FIX YOUR FEET

FIX YOUR FEET

BUILD THE BEST FOUNDATION FOR HEALTHY AND PAIN-FREE KNEES, HIPS, AND SPINE

Dr. Philip Maffetone

THE LYONS PRESS
Guilford, Connecticut

An imprint of The Globe Pequot Press

The Lyons Press is an imprint of The Globe Pequot Press.

10 9 8 7 6 5 4 3 2 1

Printed in the United States of America

Designed by Stephanie Doyle

ISBN 1-59228-198-2

Library of Congress Cataloging-in-Publication Data is available on file.

To my mother, Marjorie, who helped me with my first steps.

CONTENTS

FOREWORD

Some of what you will read in this book may run counter to conventional wisdom; but if you keep an open mind and contemplate what you read in the following pages, you will discover a new source of knowledge and a way to keep your feet working well for life.

I have benefited from Dr. Phil Maffetone's teaching for many years now. He has been an inspiration and source of knowledge in endurance training, and allowed me to compete in triathlon and stay healthy enough to complete a rigorous orthopaedic surgery residency program. During that same residency program, I completed a study on the effect of shoewear on running biomechanics, and was first inspired to design the project because of Dr. Maffetone's writings. The study won a prestigious award from an international sports medicine society, and I presented the study to favorable review at the society's international congress in Switzerland. I have also put my research to the test—running barefoot in several triathlons—and have even won my age-group.

William B. Workman, M.D.
Orthopaedic Sports Medicine Surgeon

INTRODUCTION

WHY ARE YOUR FEET IMPORTANT?

The answer to this question is simple: One pair must last a lifetime.

This is a serious book for those serious about their feet. Many of the approaches discussed here can provide quick improvements of common foot problems. However, this is not a quick-fix book. It's important to understand how your feet work if you want to truly correct and prevent future problems.

The feet are subjected to more wear and tear than any other body part. Walk a mile and you generate more than sixty tons–that's over 120,000 pounds–of stress on each foot! Fortunately, our feet are actually made to handle such natural stress. It's only when we interfere with nature that problems arise. Almost all foot problems can be prevented, and those that do arise can most often be treated conservatively through self-care. This book discusses these issues. Many foot problems, if not addressed adequately and early, can become severe enough to require professional help.

From birth until death, our feet are very important to overall health, but they may be one of the most neglected parts of the body. The feet are our structural foundation. They form the base of our body's physical stature. Any departure from optimal balance can have significant adverse effects not only locally in the feet, but above the feet in the muscles, ligaments, tendons, bones, and joints in the legs, knees, thighs, hips, pelvis, spine, and other areas, right up to our head.

These problems are often transmitted through the ankle, an extension of the upper part of the foot. Anatomists technically consider the foot and ankle as two separate parts, but in this book I will consider the ankle as a vital part of the foot for ease of discussion. The ankle is a vulnerable area; approximately twenty-five thousand people sprain an ankle each day in the United States!

Although the skeleton is an important part of our structural health, it's the skeletal muscles that allow us to move. These muscles hold up our skeleton, thus enabling it to function as a structural foundation. The early stages of most foot problems are associated with muscle imbalance.

Bony problems, including joint dysfunction, are usually secondary to muscle imbalance. Trauma can cause injury to any component of the foot, including a muscle, bone, ligament, tendon, or joint.

Another important job of the feet is to help balance the whole body. The feet continuously communicate with the brain to regulate the rest of the body's daily movements, including walking, running, and other movement. This is accomplished by powerful nerve endings at the bottom of our feet. These nerve endings are developed from infancy, and their proper function is necessary throughout our life. Disturbances of these nerve endings due to trauma, disease, poor footwear, or neglect is one common way our whole body can be adversely affected by poor foot function.

The nerve endings at the bottoms of our feet also become a potential source of powerful therapy when properly and specifically stimulated. This approach can be used both as a preventive measure and after some injury is realized.

The ability of the brain to sense the feet and in turn affect the whole body I call *foot-sense*. This important feature is discussed throughout the book.

While many problems in the body are the result of either obvious or hidden foot imbalances, some foot problems themselves are secondary to more primary disorders. When this happens, these secondary foot problems can, in turn, cause other problems.

Examples of problems that cause secondary foot dysfunction include structural faults in the spine and pelvis; muscle imbalance; trauma; shoes that don't properly fit the foot, including oversupported shoes and those with higher heels; and certain diseases such as diabetes, peripheral vascular disease, neuropathy, inflammation, and arthritis.

Foot problems are perhaps the most common type of structural injury people develop, and the most common complaint about the foot is pain. When pain presents in specific areas of the foot, it most often indicates the source of the problem. For example, pain at the top of the foot may indicate a mid-foot fracture, although there may be other causes of this type of pain. The issue of pain is discussed in later chapters in this book in terms of the different types and causes of pain and various remedies. Different types of pain control techniques are also discussed.

For most people, serious conditions in the foot are rare. However, foot problems due to less serious problems can still become debilitating: They can reduce the quality of life; lead to other areas of dysfunction such as knee, hip, or back pain; and even increase the risk of falls and other injury. The term *dysfunction,* used often in this book, refers to an area that does not work properly, typically due to some imbalance (usually muscular).

Many foot problems lead to inactivity. This may be due to foot, ankle, knee, hip, or other physical pain. Inactivity can lead to changes in metabolism, which can then lead to weight gain, circulatory insufficiency, muscle loss, poor coordination, and other more serious disabilities. Poor coordination or balance is a significant problem for those over age sixty-five.

Significant foot problems affect more than 80 percent of people over the age of sixty-five. Foot problems in these individuals dramatically increase the risk of falls. In turn, falls can reduce the quality of life and increase the risk of death as ten thousand American seniors die each year from falls. Reduced sensation of the feet, oversupported shoes, and other problems discussed in this book account for the common problem of falling.

Most shoes pose a great potential danger to the feet, much more than does the ground itself. Sports-type shoes, tight shoes, and high heels can be especially damaging due to the resulting alterations in foot function. Structurally, shoes can alter how the muscles and joints function, not only in the foot but also in areas above. Knee movement is the best example of this: With inadequate footwear, the muscles around the knee and the knee joint may move improperly. When this irregular movement continues, the result is some type of knee injury, typically resulting in pain.

In addition, shoes can alter our natural *gait*–the way we walk and run. The result is our body does not walk and run in a normal balanced way. This can lead to disability of almost any structural area of the body–from the foot itself to the head.

Rehabilitating your feet is the remedy to correct most existing problems and prevent future ones. This consists first of evaluating foot function. Understanding pain patterns, shoe wear, callous formation, and other features help determine which therapy would be most beneficial.

One of the best remedies for foot problems associated with muscle dysfunction is barefoot movement. Being barefoot should be the perfect position for the foot. This is especially true for children, whose feet have not been disturbed by shoe wear, trauma, and other wear-and-tear factors.

These and other issues are addressed in detail in the following chapters. The primary focus of this book is common foot problems rather than diseases affecting the feet. Most foot problems are of the functional type–reversible and relatively easy to correct. They are problems that can even exist without symptoms and can still cause many different problems in many other areas of the body. This book discusses the assessment and treatment of these types of problems and how to prevent them.

FIX YOUR FEET

SECTION ONE

BASIC ANATOMY

To truly understand your feet, it's important to be familiar with the basic aspects of the foot. This includes its anatomy, which comprises the bones, muscles, ligaments, tendons, and other physical aspects. The movements of the foot are also important to understand. A general comprehension of what and how things can go wrong in the foot and how to evaluate this leads to a more successful outcome. An understanding of pain is also important, as pain is part of most foot problems.

1

ANATOMY MADE SIMPLE

There's nothing simple about the human foot. It's one of the most incredible and complex bio-engineered parts of our anatomy. It combines power and speed with delicate movement and balance, solid stability with acute sensitivity, and endurance to take us almost anywhere we want to go for more than one hundred years.

This chapter offers a very simplified version of this anatomy with basic drawings showing the muscles, tendons, ligaments, and bones. There are many good textbooks, such as *Gray's Anatomy,* that detail all aspects of the foot's complex structure.

The growth of the human foot comes in spurts. During the first ten years of a child's life, foot growth averages about one-half inch a year. Between the ages of ten and twenty the yearly growth rate slows down considerably, with maturity of growth arriving between the ages of nineteen and twenty. However, the foot still gets larger with age. This is not true growth but a spreading of the foot due to metabolic changes in the body. For example, body weight, pregnancy, lifestyle, and shoe wear all could influence the foot to expand or not. Throughout life, it would not be unusual for an adult foot to increase two or more sizes during the course of normal activity. Restrictive shoes, however, can prevent this normal expansion, causing a variety of problems. At any stage of development, incorrect posture, poor walking habits, and improper footwear can also significantly disturb foot muscle function, joint alignment, and the structure of the bones themselves.

The basic anatomy of the foot, like the rest of the body, often has variations in its structures–we're not all exact replicas. But these variations are well adapted for by the muscles. The same is true between the left and right foot. Variations are common, including foot length that could vary by a whole size or more.

BONES

At birth, the bones in our feet are undeveloped–there is actually just one bone, with the rest made up of a softer material called *cartilage.* By about three years of age, much of the cartilage has become bone, and by age six all twenty-eight bones have taken shape but are still partly composed of cartilage. Even in the adult, some cartilage remains. About a quarter of the body's bones are in the feet. During this developmental stage, interfering with natural foot development can severely impact on foot function later in life.

For convenience, anatomists divide the foot into three main parts: the *forefoot, midfoot,* and *hindfoot* (see Figure 1.1). The forefoot bears half the body's weight, with the ball of the foot responsible for much of our balance.

The four smaller toes are made up of three small bones each, called *phalanges.* The big toe, called the *hallux,* has only two bones (phalanges). Under the big toe are two very small, round *sesamoid bones* within a tendon. The bones of the toes are connected to the metatarsal bones.

The midfoot has five irregularly shaped bones, which, with support from the muscles, form the foot's characteristic arches (discussed below). It is here that much of the foot's natural ability to absorb shock takes place. The bones that connect to the metatarsals are called the first, second, and third *cuneiform* bones, and the *cuboid* bone. Behind these is the *navicular* bone.

The hindfoot contains the *talus* bone (the ankle) that connects the foot to the two long bones of the leg–the smaller fibula on the outside and the tibia, the main leg bone. The talus bone is also connected to and rests on the *calcaneous* bone (the heel), the largest bone of the foot, which assists in stability during movement and standing. In the back of the foot, the Achilles tendon supports the calcaneous bone. Figure 1.2 also shows a front view of the ankle.

In some individuals, small extra bones called *accessory ossicles* may exist throughout the foot. In

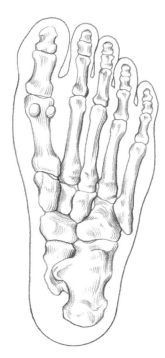

FIGURE 1.1 View of the bones from the bottom of the foot.

addition, there may be extra sesamoid bones. When present, these extra bones don't inherently pose any particular problem.

JOINTS

When two bones come together they form a *joint,* which allows smooth movement between the bones (see Figure 1.3). Each bone has softer *articular cartilage* at its end for protection. A type of cover, known as the *articular capsule,* which contains a thick lubricating liquid called *synovial fluid,* surrounds joints. The joints and cartilage cushion the bones and protect them from making direct contact.

Together with the ankle, the foot has some thirty-three joints. Coordination occurs with the help of more than one hundred *ligaments,* which connect bones to other bones, with *tendons* (which connect muscles to bones), and with muscles. The bones provide a solid foundation and leverage for muscles to move the body.

MUSCLES

The feet are our physical foundation. More than thirty muscles and tendons of the foot provide a certain range of motion and stability not only to the foot itself, but also indirectly to the whole body. The muscles give the foot its shape by holding the bones in position. Without muscle support, the skeleton and all its bones would collapse. Much of the foot support comes from muscles that attach higher up in the leg, with tendons coming down into and attaching on bones of the foot. Many other muscles are exclusively found within the foot itself.

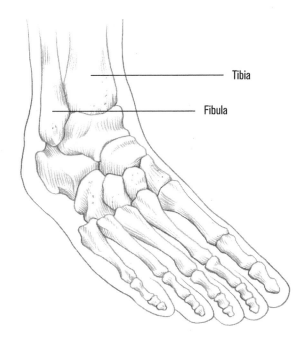

FIGURE 1.2 Front view of the ankle showing the leg bones—tibia and fibula—that attach to the foot.

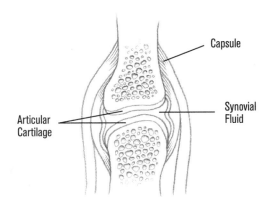

FIGURE 1.3 Cross section of a joint with articular cartilage, capsule and synovial fluid.

All the muscles of the foot, ankle, and leg play a vital role in foot movement, or *mechanics*. Because of the extensive nature of the structure and function of all these muscles, this discussion will be limited to only the most important muscles and muscle groups. Figures 1.4, a, b, and c show the muscles discussed below.

FIGURES 1.4 Some of the muscles of the leg, ankle, and foot (a): tibialis posterior (not visible—covered by other muscles), gastrocnemius, soleus; (b): tibialis anterior, peroneus longus and brevis, peroneus tertius; (c): plantar muscles of the foot.

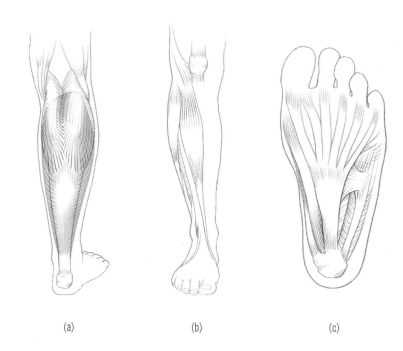

(a)   (b)   (c)

Tibialis Posterior

The *tibialis posterior* is a long muscle that attaches to the two leg bones—the tibia and fibula—in the middle of the back calf under the large *gastrocnemius* and *soleus* muscles. The tibialis posterior muscle runs down the back of the leg around the inside of the ankle (the *medial* side) and into the bottom of foot, inserting into different bones. Contracting this muscle allows you to point your foot down (an action called *plantar flexion*). It also turns the foot inward. The ability to rise on your toes requires the function of the tibialis posterior muscle.

The tibialis posterior is one of the most important muscles associated with many foot, ankle, and knee problems. It's a key stabilizing muscle for both the midfoot and hindfoot. When this muscle does not work properly, it can cause a variety of nonspecific symptoms that are difficult to diagnose.

Because of its importance in supporting the medial arch (discussed below), *inhibition* or "weakness" of this muscle, perhaps its most common problem, causes poor arch support that can lead to excess pronation and other problems. Secondary to tibialis posterior inhibition is often tightness of the gastrocnemius and soleus muscles, and sometimes pain in the Achilles tendon. Abnormal muscle inhibition, as discussed throughout this book, is a condition similar to a weak muscle.

TIBIALIS ANTERIOR

The *tibialis anterior* is also a long muscle that attaches predominantly on the upper half of the tibia in the front of the leg (and slightly to the outside), where it is easily felt as a relatively large mass. It runs downward and becomes a large tendon, which is easily visible when lifting the foot just above the ankle. It continues down across the ankle and attaches into the first metatarsal bone and the first cuneform bone.

The tibialis anterior muscle raises the foot upward (an action called *dorsal flexion*) and assists in turning the foot inward. When inhibited, it can cause instability of the ankle just like the tibialis posterior, may be responsible for problems in the first metatarsal joint, and can cause so-called shinsplints.

PERONEUS MUSCLES

The *peroneus longus* and *brevis* muscles attach mostly on the fibula on the outside, or *lateral side* of the leg, with some parts attached to the tibia. These muscles turn to tendon right above the ankle and can be seen just behind the bony end of the fibula (called the *lateral malleolus*) where it attaches to the ankle. The longus portion of the peroneus attaches into the cuneform bone and first metatarsal bone, with the brevis attaching to the fifth metatarsal bone.

The peroneus longus and brevis muscles stabilize the outside, or *lateral* portion of the ankle, allowing the foot to elevate or *evert* while the ankle is *plantar flexed* (foot pointed down). If you try to contract this muscle by pointing your foot down and out, you can easily see and feel it on the outside of the leg.

The *peroneus tertius* muscle is a much shorter but important muscle that also stabilizes the outside of the ankle. This muscle attaches on the lower portion of the fibula bone on the outside of the ankle and inserts into the fifth metatarsal bone. It allows the outside of the foot to turn upward with the ankle. This muscle is often involved in common ankle sprains, and if it does not heal properly after trauma, it can contribute to chronic ankle problems.

Gastrocnemius and Soleus

The bulk of calf muscle on the back of the leg is made up of the gastrocnemius and soleus muscles. Together, these two muscles are sometimes referred to as the *triceps surae.* They attach into the upper leg bones and, in part, above the knee into the back of the thighbone, the *femur.* These muscles are the main foot extenders, important for rising on our toes during any movement. These two muscles form the Achilles tendon beginning at about the middle of the calf. This tendon runs downward and attaches into the back of the calcaneus bone. Both the muscles and the Achilles tendon provide great support for the foot through stability of the heel.

Plantar Muscles

There are four layers of muscles on the bottom of the foot consisting of a dozen separate muscles. Overall, these muscles have grabbing actions important for walking, running, foot coordination, and balance. These actions are best observed when barefoot. Wearing shoes can render these and other foot muscles less active and could lead to chronic foot problems.

Foot Arches

As a means of supporting the weight of the body, for shock absorption, and for propulsion, the bottom of the foot is constructed of a serious of arches. These arches also allow the foot to adapt to uneven surfaces. The muscles are the key factor in supporting the arches, and maintaining them is vital for normal foot function. Figure 1.5 shows the main arch, but this drawing may be misleading because without muscle support, the foot collapses and there are no arches. Interfering with the normal function of the arches, most often by disturbing the natural action of the muscles that support them, is a common cause of injury and chronic foot problems.

FIGURES 1.5 Medial arch of the foot without muscle support.

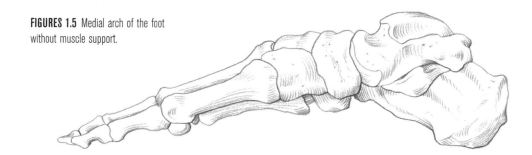

The *medial arch* is one of the two large arches and is the one familiar to most people. It runs along the inner aspect of the bottom of the foot. The side view of the bones of the foot (without supporting muscles) in Figure 1.5 clearly shows the magnitude of the medial arch. This arch is maintained by the action of muscles, especially the tibialis posterior.

The *lateral longitudinal arch* is the second-largest arch and runs along the outside of the bottom of the foot. The *transverse* or *metatarsal arches* are in the midfoot across the ball of the foot, and the *short longitudinal arches* are in the hindfoot. The peroneus longus and brevis and the plantar muscles on the bottom of the foot support these arches.

OTHER IMPORTANT STRUCTURES

Many other structures in the foot support its actions and maintain foot health. These include fascia, nerves, skin, and blood vessels.

FASCIA

Throughout the foot and ankle thin fibrous sheaths called *fascia* provide great strength. This material helps stabilize the foot, especially in areas of the joints, and helps bind the tendons, which aid the muscles in their supporting efforts. The fascia blends with many other soft tissues of the foot and ankle. Important fascia is found on the top of the foot (the *dorsal fascia*), on the bottom of the foot (the *plantar fascia*), and around the ankle.

NERVES

Within the muscles, tendons, ligaments, joints, and other soft tissues of the foot are important nerve endings that sense all movement, pressure, and body position. This information is sent to the central nervous system (spinal cord and brain) so we can respond appropriately to activity of the foot—a process I refer to as *foot-sense*. Next to the spine, the foot has more nerve activity than any other region of the body.

We're familiar with our senses of smell, taste, and sight, but foot-sense, though not as well known, is equally important. For example, if we step on a pebble while barefoot we react immediately by contracting certain muscles that lift our foot off the pebble. More commonly, we don't have to look to see the position of our foot because we "sense" its location. The same is true with our sense of movement—we don't have to look at each footstep we take to walk effectively. Foot-sense can also be observed while balancing on one foot. The brain interprets incoming messages from the foot we're balancing on and sends back messages to muscles throughout the body to continuously adjust our posture to keep from falling. These movements may include tilting the head, moving the arms up and down, or whatever is necessary to keep balanced. Without effective foot-sense, proper balance could not occur.

Foot-sense is a vital function for foot stability, to prevent injury, and to recover from an injury. Imbalanced muscles, overuse, disease, and many types of shoes can cause the nervous system to have poor foot-sense, leading to vulnerability for injury and other problems. With poor foot-sense comes a response from the brain to body muscles that may not be correct. The result is the body does not properly compensate for even a minor foot problem, ultimately leading to an injury or worsening of an existing problem.

Because the nerves in the feet significantly affect balance, restoring normal movement and posture, even for brief periods, can be very therapeutic. This is a key benefit of being barefoot–the most natural of all positions for the foot. Improving foot-sense in the feet can be done with almost anyone and at any age.

Pain is also relayed from the feet to the brain through nerves. Pain fibers are located in most structures of the foot, including the covering of the bones. During injury, the intensity of the pain does not necessarily relate to the severity of injury, as sometimes a relatively minor injury can elicit great pain because of the sensitivity of the foot.

SKIN, NAILS, AND BLOOD VESSELS

The skin is obviously important for normal foot function. It protects the structures inside the foot, is an important site for nerve endings, and cushions the foot with the help of a fat pad under the *calcaneal* (heel) bone.

The skin contains many nerve endings for foot-sense, especially on the bottom of the foot. The skin on the feet is very durable, especially on the sole, and can withstand many more pounds of force compared to the hand and fingers before it is cut open. When the skin is subject to chronic stress, such as excessive wear and tear, the skin thickens, resulting in *calluses*.

Calluses generally are almost always caused by shoes and can be secondary to toe deformities such as a hammertoe or bunion. They typically occur over a bony prominence. A callus that forms on a toe is called a *corn*. Calluses are usually not painful, except certain types that are typically on the bottom of the foot. These may be *plantar keratoses*, or seed calluses, and are very small. Some calluses cause sufficient pressure on the metatarsal joints to cause pain in the joint.

Calluses can usually be differentiated from warts by pinching both sides together–warts are generally tender and calluses are usually not, with the rare exception noted above.

Toenails are adversely affected by trauma, most often by shoes. An ingrown toenail usually occurs in the big toe due to either poor fitting shoes or improper nail trimming, or both. This problem can lead to fungal or bacterial infections (see Chapter 15).

Another problem found in toenails is the so-called blackened nail, which results from trauma directly on the nail and is most often caused by shoes. A darkened toenail usually means the shoe is too small or otherwise not fitting the foot. Some dark toenails are due to fungal infections.

Blood vessels in the foot are very important to maintain the health of all the structures we've discussed. The arteries bring nutrient-rich blood into the foot in the form of glucose, fat, protein, vitamins, minerals, and other essential elements, including oxygen. The veins carry blood back to the heart and remove carbon dioxide, excess water, and waste products from the foot. Poor blood flow due to inactivity, poor muscle function, or abnormally narrowed or closed blood vessels can cause or aggravate existing foot problems from within. Improper blood flow can also cause skin ulceration, which is common in diabetics.

When all the important components of the foot and ankle function properly, movement is most efficient. The next chapter discusses the normal movements of the foot and ankle.

2

FOOT POSTURE
AND MOVEMENT

Optimal foot posture and movement is associated with normal foot function. Given a relatively normal foot (one that's not deformed), its posture and movement is greatly dependent upon balanced muscles. For example, the structures above a normal foot may not be balanced and can lead to the potential of abnormal foot function. This can occur if the muscles in or around the pelvis are not balanced; the hip, thigh, and leg could rotate excessively during movement causing the foot to bear weight in an abnormal fashion. Ultimately, this can cause a secondary foot problem.

When our feet are balanced, our movement, whether walking, running, or involved in some other locomotion, is accomplished most efficiently. This means wear and tear is minimal, as is the energy requirement. Any deviation from normal regarding posture and movement causes more wear and tear not only in the foot, but also in the ankle, knee, hip, pelvis, spine, and other areas. It causes us to expend more energy on movement, too—in some cases a significant amount more. Those with a relatively minor foot problem that causes a change in the way they move can waste a significant amount of energy in accomplishing the same task. Even the weight of light shoes causes us to expend more energy, with larger and heavier shoes using up yet more.

Like other structures in the body, foot movement occurs when a muscle or muscles contract, pulling on a tendon or tendons that pull a bone or bones in the same direction. The joint(s) and ligament(s) between the bones allow a certain amount of movement, with ligaments, joints, fascia, and opposing muscles preventing excess movement that would cause injury.

The weight of the body itself on the foot also causes movement—even standing still is accompanied by subtle sways—with the muscles playing a key role in supporting these weight-bearing actions. In addition, standing still requires significant contraction on the part of some muscles to maintain the foot stability that holds us up.

The body is a complex *biomechanical kinetic chain* where all movements are precisely related. An abnormal movement in one area can interfere with proper movements at other joints. Abnormal foot movement, for example, could force a variety of muscles to compensate, causing adaptation in the ankle and knee, which in turn causes both joints and related muscles to move abnormally. When foot imbalance is present, there can be a negative impact on the knees, hips, pelvis, and spine and even on areas such as the shoulders and into the head. This scenario is a common cause of aches and pains, some serious, above the foot and ankle.

NORMAL FOOT MOTIONS

The foot has a variety of normal movements. The toes can *flex*, which curls them downward, and *extend*, bringing them upward. They have slight movement from side to side—seen in spreading the toes and squeezing them together. These actions can make very good exercises for those who need to rehabilitate their foot muscles (discussed in Chapter 11). If you're unable to squeeze or spread your toes, it may indicate poor muscle function, and only rarely more serious problems.

INVERSION AND EVERSION

The foot can rotate inward and outward. The inward rotation is called *inversion* and results in the sole of the foot turning inward (see Figure 2.1b). The muscles that accomplish this are the tibialis posterior and anterior. The outward rotation is called *eversion* with the sole of the foot turned out. The muscles responsible for eversion include the peroneus longus and brevis, with some action from the peroneus tertius (see Figure 2.1a).

The movement of inversion and eversion takes place in the joints between the talus and calcaneus bones. Pain during these specific movements may indicate a problem with the talus and the muscles that support it, typically the tibialis posterior and sometimes tibialis anterior.

GAIT

The act of moving, such as walking or running, is termed *gait*. During different types or styles of normal gaits, the stress on the feet can vary, which our feet are made to endure. The full phase of a normal gait includes the point our heel strikes the ground, through rolling our foot forward, to lifting and pushing off our toes, to swinging our foot forward to strike the ground again (see Figure 2.2, a, b, c). During this normal gait, the foot makes many adaptations. It can effectively adjust to any uneven surface, become rigid enough to propel itself and roll over the big toe, go through various ranges of motion, and effectively absorb shock. This is accomplished by the actions of muscles, ligaments, tendons, fascia, and bones.

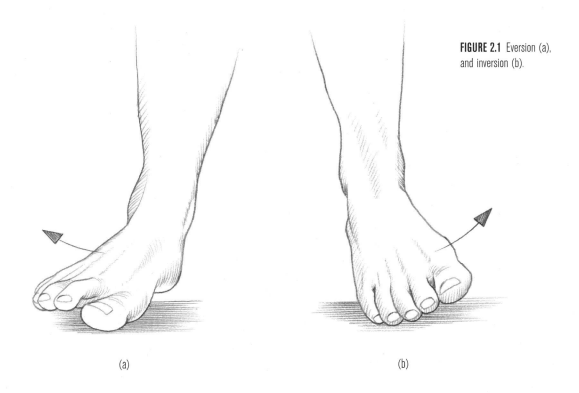

FIGURE 2.1 Eversion (a), and inversion (b).

(a)   (b)

A certain amount of energy is required to propel the body, with more needed for running or other higher intensity activity compared to walking. This energy comes from two separate but important sources. First, the muscles create energy from within, using both glucose (sugar) and fat as fuel. Second, the gravitational energy from the force of each foot's impact with the ground during movement is absorbed into the muscles and tendons and recycled back to assist in movement. Walking and running in soft sand, for example, is more difficult because there is considerably less impact energy to reuse for propulsion.

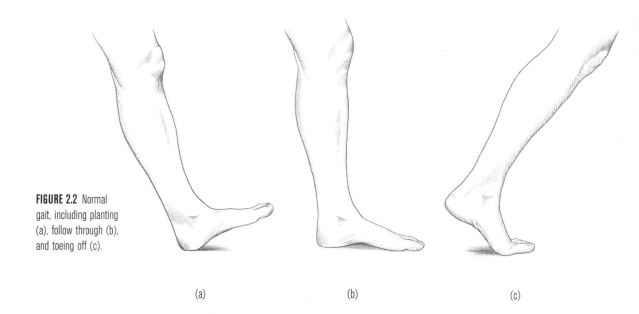

FIGURE 2.2 Normal gait, including planting (a), follow through (b), and toeing off (c).

(a)   (b)   (c)

Pronation and Supination

During a normal gait, *pronation* and *supination* occur in the foot. Pronation is very important for shock absorption. During heel strike, the foot begins to roll inward, it everts slightly, and the arch flattens. This process is called pronation. It is a normal action that takes place in every step in every healthy foot. The purpose of this is to loosen the foot so it can adapt to the surface, especially in the event of uneven terrain.

Following pronation, as the foot continues through its gait, supination occurs. First the foot turns outward, then it changes from a flexible foot to become rigid so it can propel the foot and push off. During this phase the foot inverts slightly and the arches get higher, enabling the foot to properly roll over the big toe. Figure 2.3, a, b, c, shows these actions.

A number of factors can disrupt a person's normal gait. These include muscle imbalance in the foot or areas above, such as the pelvis or spine, which influences foot function. In addition, injury, pain, and diseases that affect blood flow, cause inflammation, or disturb muscle function in the foot can disturb gait.

The most common factor that changes a normal gait to an abnormal one is wearing shoes. Most shoes, including the sports type such as the popular running shoes, change the gait by causing the stride length to be abnormally longer. This results in an abnormal heel strike–hitting the ground farther back on the heel. This is especially a problem when jogging or running because it places more shock through the foot and into the knee and occurs despite the shoe cushioning or other shoe designs. Barefoot movement of any type does not cause the same stress.

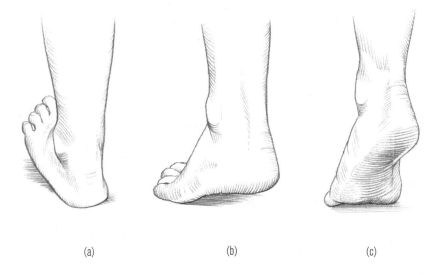

(a) (b) (c)

FIGURE 2.3 The action of pronation and supination. At the point of heel strike (a) and follow-through (b) the foot pronates, with supination occurring in the toe-off (c).

The notion that some people are "pronators" while others are "supinators" is a gross oversimplification that is often presented to an unsuspecting public. That shoe companies make special shoes for one group or the other is an example of marketing hype. We all pronate and supinate. The reason some people excessively pronate or supinate is more often from wearing shoes, especially when it comes to children, whose feet need to properly develop without shoes.

In all, our feet were made for walking, running, hopping, jumping, and all other natural movements. When we interfere with our natural movement, such as when we wear shoes, problems can arise. Apart from sandals and moccasins, humans evolved barefoot–for millions of years our feet were free. Suddenly, in only the past few hundred years, shoes of many types have restricted our feet, disturbed our gait, and caused untold problems to our feet, triggering other problems throughout the body they support.

In one sense, the foot is a highly complex structure with even more intricate function that scientists continue to unravel and understand. However, the awareness that the foot is a perfectly made natural part of our anatomy and can function just fine on its own will help in our appreciation of this structure and in our ability to prevent and correct most problems we inflict upon it. The two main types of foot problems we encounter are described in the next chapter.

3

TWO TYPES OF FOOT PROBLEMS

In a very general sense, there are only two broad types of foot problems. The first are those that don't elicit pain or other obvious dysfunction but are silent in their impairment. I have termed these silent foot conditions *asymptomatic foot problems*. The second type includes those that produce pain and obvious disability. We'll call these *symptomatic foot problems*. Most foot problems are silent and, therefore, fall into the first category. These asymptomatic problems are due mostly to relatively minor muscle imbalance. While these problems may come and go without notice, they can also be the cause of the majority of secondary problems producing pain and disability.

ASYMPTOMATIC FOOT PROBLEMS

There are a variety of types of asymptomatic foot problems. Most are due to subtle muscle imbalances in the foot, although muscle imbalances in the leg, pelvis, or spine can also contribute. Almost everyone has subtle muscle imbalance due to the everyday wear and tear of normal movement. It's like doing spring yard work or cleaning out your basement—you're bound to get some bumps and bruises from wear and tear, but you'll heal up quickly.

Most of this wear and tear in the foot is corrected through the body's natural ability to fix many of its own problems. However, sometimes the body does not correct these problems and they become chronic. When this happens, a significant imbalance can occur leading to symptomatic foot problems. Let's look at one example of how this can happen.

Perhaps during the course of a hectic day at work, you quickly turn your foot, not enough to sprain it, or even remember it happened, but sufficiently to *overstretch* your tibialis posterior muscle. This relatively small muscle attaches into the leg bones–the tibia and fibula–in the middle of the back calf under the large gastrocnemius and soleus muscles. It runs down the back of the leg around the ankle and inserts into bones in the bottom of the foot.

At first you don't notice anything different. It's a silent "injury" that may have corrected itself after a few days, just like a minor bruise or cut. But on this occasion, the muscle remained sprained, in other words, overstretched. When muscles overstretch, they become weaker and inhibited and less effective at their normal tasks. The tibialis posterior muscle helps support many structures, including the medial arch. Without this support normal pronation cannot occur and excess pronation takes place. You may remain in this state of imbalance for days or weeks, or even months or years, before feeling anything different.

In this scenario, the problem now begins a domino effect: The gastrocnemius and soleus muscles tighten as a normal compensation, and for the first time you feel some slight discomfort in your calf. You don't realize that your medial arch is not functioning normally and weight bearing is abnormal. It's now more than a month after the initial incident, and for the first time you begin to feel some discomfort in your knee. After another month, the knee is causing pain, especially during walking.

Any successful remedy would have to include correction of the tibialis posterior muscle. The body may be able to correct this on its own, but often if the problem becomes chronic this may not happen. Sometimes rest will allow this to happen, although sometimes rest can make problems worse.

MUSCLE INHIBITION

Muscle problems like the one just described are common causes of many foot problems. The most common type of muscle problem is the so-called "weak" muscle. This is not a weakness due to inactivity or lack of use (although this is also a problem common in people who are very inactive). In this case, it is technically called an abnormal *muscle inhibition.*

Muscle inhibition in itself may not be a problem, except when it's not normal. Muscles normally "turn on" and "turn off" as we move–referred to as *facilitation* and *inhibition,* respectively. Normally, while one muscle is facilitated and contracts, another is inhibited and becomes lax. This is associated with normal body movement. But when a muscle becomes inhibited when it's not supposed to, it is an abnormal situation. In this instance, the inhibited muscle is lax, elongated, "turned off," over-stretched, and does not function properly. The tibialis posterior muscle described above was an example of how an inhibited muscle can cause a problem elsewhere.

Most abnormal muscle inhibition typically leads to secondary muscle tightness, or *overfacilitation*. In most cases, the muscle that is inhibited is asymptomatic but the secondary muscle overfacilitation is felt as tightness. In some cases, this pattern of abnormal inhibition and secondary tightness (or abnormal facilitation)—referred to as muscle im-balance—causes a joint to move abnormally. This could produce symptoms in the joint—typically just discomfort but sometimes pain. This now becomes a symptomatic problem, which is discussed later in this chapter.

Muscle inhibition can often arise from trauma. A sprained ankle is a common example of a trauma that causes a gross overstretching of muscles. Other trauma can do the same, such as a blow directly to the muscle. Even minor trauma such as regular wear and tear or minor repetitive stress can sometimes cause muscle inhibition. Repetitive stress includes any regular motion such as cycling, walking, jogging, running, and so forth.

Many different types of footwear can cause muscles to become in-hibited. Oversupported shoes, sports shoes that are too soft, and dress shoes with higher heels are common examples. Wearing shoes that don't fit properly can also cause muscle inhibition. In addition, sup-ports such as orthotics, braces, arch supports, and other devices can sometimes cause muscle inhibition, especially if the supports don't precisely match the foot or if the support is used for too long a period. These and other issues regarding shoes and supports are discussed in Section II: Shoes.

Improper stretching routines can cause muscle inhibition. Many people think stretching is a healthy practice, which it can be if per-formed correctly. But in many cases, stretching is too aggressive, im-properly performed, or excessive ranges of motion are obtained with unhealthy consequences. One is that muscles are overstretched and thus become abnormally inhibited.

To summarize, some potential causes of muscle inhibition include the following:

- Trauma (macro or micro)
- Wear and tear
- Repetitive stress
- Improper shoes

- Improper supports
- Overstretching

Correction of muscle inhibition is discussed in Section III: Treatment. The full spectrum of muscle problems, including inhibition, is discussed in the next chapter.

REDUCED FOOT-SENSE

Another type of asymptomatic foot problem is the loss of foot-sense—the body's inability to sense properly the ground through the nerve endings on the bottom of the foot—during the aging process. Some mistakenly refer to this as part of the "normal" aging process. However, this is most often a case of inactivity. In those individuals who regularly use their feet through exercise and other activity, age-related loss of foot-sense need not be a problem. Active individuals maintain much of their normal foot function throughout their lives.

Reduced sensation from the feet can be conscious, but it's more often a subconscious problem leading to loss of balance. The risk of falls is very high in those with reduced foot-sense. Falls lead to significant reductions in quality of life as many have long hospital stays and rehabilitation may not be highly successful. The result is a further reduction in activity, often complete inactivity. In those who remain active, the incidence of another fall is great.

Worse is the issue of mortality from falls. Two-thirds or more of accidental deaths in those aged sixty-five and over may be associated with falls. About a third or more of those who fall and fracture their femur bone, including the hip, die within one year.

Reduced sensation from the feet not only occurs in the elderly, but studies now show that even young athletes can have significantly reduced foot-sense due to the use of thick soled and oversupported sports shoes. This could not only adversely affect daily movements, which are vital in sports, but increase the injury rate as well. This issue is further addressed in Chapters 7 and 8.

SYMPTOMATIC FOOT PROBLEMS

Common problems in the foot produce signs and symptoms ranging from pain, swelling, and localized tenderness, to numbness or tingling, weakness, and reduced range of motion in the form of stiffness or reduced movement. These symptoms indicate that some aspect of the foot and ankle is not working properly and may even lead to further problems.

Symptomatic problems are usually obvious and may be due to a variety of causes, including three common ones: chronic muscle inhibition, trauma, and disease.

CHRONIC MUSCLE INHIBITION

An asymptomatic muscle inhibition can eventually cause foot pain, injury, or other problems. This is a very common reason for symptomatic foot problems. In fact, this may be the most common cause of symptomatic foot problems.

Obvious symptomatic foot problems may develop suddenly, and others more slowly over a period of time beginning with only the slightest clue. In either case, they may also disappear the same way, as do many symptomatic foot problems. This happens because other muscles may compensate for them. In some of these cases, the compensation itself–specifically, the muscle involved in compensating–can cause other symptoms. This is part of the domino effect described above. It can occur with any group of muscles in the foot, ankle, leg, or above.

Sometimes, muscle compensation can even shift to the other side of the body. For example, a chronic muscle inhibition in the right foot may cause the body to shift weight bearing, putting excess weight through the left foot, with an eventual problem created there. In the end, it will be the left foot–opposite the side of the primary problem–that produces the symptoms.

Chronic muscle inhibition also results in muscle tightness, or overfacilitation. Tight calf muscles, tight plantar muscles (the bottom of the foot), or tightness in the front of the leg are common complaints that are often secondary to primary muscle inhibitions. The symptoms for these conditions are often described as Achilles tendonitis, plantar fasciitis, or shinsplints, respectively.

TRAUMA

While relatively minor traumas may cause muscle inhibition, more serious trauma can cause fracture, serious laceration, or crushing injury. These and others are some common examples of traumatic causes of foot problems. Even more common are ankle sprains. Ankle sprains are often due to foot dysfunction, which is typically aggravated by improper footwear such as thick-soled sports shoes or high-top sneakers. This issue is discussed in depth in Section II: Shoes.

Whatever the cause of the trauma, it often results in abnormal muscle inhibition. In a sprained ankle, for example, the trauma damages the muscles along with other important foot structures such as ligaments, tendons, fascia, or even blood vessels. An ankle sprain typically includes damage to the lateral collateral ligaments, but at other times different structures may be damaged such as the peroneal tendon, local joints or bones, or even nerves. But in almost all cases, muscle inhibition occurs as well, and many of these muscles stay chronically inhibited, slowing recovery time, maintaining pain, and often allowing a recurrence of ankle sprain. In fact, the majority of those who sprain their ankle will do so again. This is especially true for athletes.

Trauma induces muscle inhibition in most cases. Pain that does not diminish or is almost eliminated within a few days of injury may also be associated with muscle inhibition that has not been corrected or compensated for by the body. Many traumatic injuries will recover significantly faster when normal muscle function is restored as quickly as possible.

Disease

Among the common diseases that cause foot problems are diabetes (types 1 and 2), vascular (blood vessel) disease, neuropathy (nerve damage), rheumatoid arthritis, and other inflammatory conditions. In many patients, these problems can overlap. They are systemic, or systemwide problems, not just ones related to the feet.

In diabetes, there are many adverse changes that take place, especially in those who don't address their health needs adequately by eating right and exercising. Problems can occur in the nerves of the leg, ankle, and foot causing loss of nerve function, including sensation. The structure of the foot and ankle are affected, including bones, joints, and muscles. This neuropathy has an adverse effect on movement, which worsens an already poor circulation (reduced blood flow). Combined with lowered immunity, the result may be poor wound healing, infection, and ulceration.

Chronic inflammation is a common problem associated with most chronic diseases and typically precedes the disease. Like rheumatoid arthritis, inflammation is a systemwide problem that also affects the foot.

Whether you have an asymptomatic foot problem or one that is giving you symptoms, the first step in correcting the problem is assessment—the subject of the next chapter.

4

ASSESSING YOUR FEET

If your foot does not function like it should, the first step should be a foot assessment. The term *assessment* refers to an evaluation or appraisal. Through an evaluation process, much like Sherlock Holmes would follow, you can arrive at the cause of the problem, or at least, how to fix it.

Assessment is not *diagnosis*. Most foot problems have no diagnosis. A diagnosis pertains to disease or serious conditions such as a fracture. Most foot problems are *functional* in nature and are without disease or serious disorders. In other words, they are *dysfunctions*. Assessment involves evaluating a foot's function.

A muscle imbalance is an example of a common dysfunction and a simple statement suggesting the cause of a particular complaint. An assessment may not result in a diagnosis because most foot problems are not associated with serious conditions. An assessment is a gathering of important information about the foot and its function.

Assessment is very important because only after an adequate assessment can a successful therapy be applied. Otherwise, any therapy is just a guess. The most successful therapies are the ones that most appropriately match the specific problem and those that treat its cause. To find this match, an assessment is necessary.

As assessment can come in the form of questions, such as the ones discussed below, a history, or other clues, often using signs and symptoms as a guide.

In the process of assessing your foot, a variety of indications may be present. These take the form of *signs* and *symptoms*. Signs are more objective indications such as skin rash, swelling, or the results from an X ray demonstrating a broken bone. The wear patterns on your shoes and your footprints in the sand are other examples of signs.

Symptoms are more elusive and difficult to measure objectively, which is not to say that they are less important as they are often clues to the cause of the problem. Pain may be the most common of all symptoms, and there are different forms of pain, as discussed in Chapter 5. Feelings of weakness, imbalance, or "it just doesn't feel right" are other examples of common symptoms people describe.

Some foot problems are *acute,* meaning they are a recent occurrence, taking place within two weeks. Problems referred to as *chronic* have been present for a longer period, including recurrent problems such as a chronic ankle sprain. These are more than two weeks old.

Overall, most foot problems are directly or indirectly due to muscle imbalance. Even in cases of trauma or fracture, muscle imbalance plays a key role. Muscle imbalance can make the foot vulnerable to sprains, or secondary muscle imbalance can occur after a traumatic injury, including fracture, which can impair recovery.

MUSCLE IMBALANCE

This section reviews some of the points made about muscle function from previous chapters and expands the discussion to incorporate the full spectrum of muscle function.

Muscles move bones and allow us to move our feet, which in turn allow for body locomotion. Muscles can and will take on many different degrees of function and dysfunction. In general, the full spectrum of muscle function can range from very loose muscles (gross weakness) to true spastic muscles. Within these two extremes are a number of other important states, some normal and others not. These include abnormal inhibition and facilitation, and normal muscle function. Figure 4.1 shows these muscle functions.

FIGURE 4.1

Very Loose <---> Very Tight					
Weak	Abnormal inhibition	Normal inhibition	Normal facilitation	Abnormal facilitation	Spasm
------ abnormal ------ function		------ normal ------ function		------ abnormal ------ function	

GROSS MUSCLE WEAKNESS

On one end of the spectrum is gross muscle weakness. This is usually the result of long-term inactivity (such as bed rest or restriction to a wheelchair), physical muscle loss (due to poor nutrition, poor aging, or disease), or nerve damage (which can occur after a stroke or spinal cord injury). Gross muscle weakness is often due to combinations of problems. For example, insufficient activity and low dietary protein in many elderly people result in significant muscle loss leading to gross muscle weakness.

These weak muscles have little if any ability to work, being totally or nearly totally dysfunctional. These types of problems usually require help from a professional to rehabilitate the muscle or muscles. In some cases, 100 percent recovery is not possible. However, when the correct approach is taken, even chronic gross muscle weakness can sometimes be restored to more normal function.

ABNORMAL MUSCLE INHIBITION

Less serious but potentially the cause of most foot problems are abnormally inhibited muscles. These muscles usually have some function, but not sufficient activity to prevent the problems they create. They have the ability to function normally but are "turned off" due to a variety of problems such as trauma, blood flow, nerve disturbance, or others, including a combination of causes that are not permanent.

Abnormal muscle inhibition is usually primary to muscle tightness. The combination of muscle inhibition and muscle tightness results in muscle imbalance. Sometimes the body corrects these inhibited muscles, and at other times some common remedies may correct them. Stretching a muscle with this type of problem can make it worse, as an inhibited muscle is already overstretched.

Abnormal muscle inhibition may involve a single muscle but more often there is more than one muscle involved. When the problem becomes chronic the help of a professional may be required. Certain professionals perform manual muscle testing to determine which muscles may be abnormally inhibited.

NORMAL MUSCLE INHIBITION AND FACILITATION

During normal gait, certain muscles are contracted, or *facilitated*, while others are relaxed or *inhibited*. An example of this is when we are taking a step forward. When our foot is moving forward and pulled upward, the tibialis anterior muscle is facilitated. At the same time, the opposite muscles, including the gastrocnemius and soleus, are inhibited or relaxed. After the foot hits the ground and rolls forward, the act of toeing off creates an opposite action–tibialis anterior inhibition and gastrocnemius and soleus facilitation.

ABNORMAL MUSCLE FACILITATION

Muscles that remain too contracted are *abnormally facilitated*. This condition is more often secondary to a primary abnormal muscle inhibition. The most common example is a tight gastrocnemius and soleus secondary to an abnormal inhibition of the tibialis posterior muscles. This problem is sensed as tightness and is the reason many people stretch abnormally facilitated muscles. This often does not solve the problem and sometimes makes it worse long-term as abnormally inhibited muscles are often stretched in the process. Abnormal muscle facilitation may involve a single muscle, but more often there is more than one muscle involved.

MUSCLE CRAMP

A muscle cramp is a stronger, sudden muscle contraction that involves overfacilitation. It usually occurs during activity, but waking in the middle of the night with foot or leg cramps is not uncommon. The cause of muscle cramps is not known and may be very individual (one person's cramp may be caused by something different than another person's cramp). A muscle cramp is often a single muscle or muscle group. Possible causes include dehydration, low levels of sodium or magnesium, an overworked muscle, or a drug side effect. Muscle cramps generally last a relatively short time (unless you're having a bad one; then it feels like a long time). The terms *muscle cramps* and *spasms* are often used interchangeably as their definitions are somewhat scant.

MUSCLE SPASM

True muscle spasms are not common. They are a more severe form of muscle tightness that is usually constant and occurs most often in people with neurological diseases, such as multiple sclerosis and cerebral palsy and those with severe spinal cord injury. A neurologic disorder causing a primary muscle spasm often creates a secondary muscle inhibition. The result is significant loss of motion and poor gait.

None of the above muscle problems can be assessed using X ray. Gross muscle weakness can be observed as dysfunction by watching the person as he or she tries to walk or by manual muscle testing. In the case of abnormal muscle inhibition, the problem can be assessed using postural analysis and very specific manual muscle testing. In the case of an abnormally facilitated muscle, it often gives a symptom of tightness, although sometimes this is very subtle. In many cases cramps or spasms can be *palpated*–or felt by the fingertips as very hard muscles. Severe restriction of movement is also associated with muscle spasm.

In some situations, the electrical activity of the muscle can be tested using an electromyographic device (EMG). In gross muscle weakness, biofeedback that incorporates EMG can be very successful.

MUSCLE STRENGTH AND POWER

None of our discussion thus far has focused on muscle *strength* and *power*. Muscle strength is the maximum force generated by the muscle. In other words, strength is the maximum weight a person can lift at one time. The definition of power includes a time component: Power is the combination of strength and speed of the movement.

Most of our discussions in this book will focus on muscle function and balance, which relate to the normal movement of the muscle and appropriate balance of facilitation and inhibition, regardless of strength and power. A muscle that functions well may have a high or low level of power or strength. Even a very powerful weight lifter can have muscle inhibition, and the most frail and out-of-shape elderly person has muscle facilitation. In almost all foot problems, strength and power are not a factor when it comes to injury.

HOW TO MAKE AN ASSESSMENT

The first question to ask about a foot problem is how it happened. This is referred to as a *history*. Perhaps the first question should be, what caused the problem? If it was trauma—a twisted ankle, a fall down the stairs, a heavy object falling on it—that answers one big question. If there was trauma, ruling out a fracture is important, as discussed later in this chapter. If the problem began soon after you started wearing a new pair of shoes, it may mean the obvious: that those shoes may not properly match your feet. Or, perhaps the problem coincided with a new or modification in your exercise routine. Increased use of your feet may cause symptoms in a foot with asymptomatic problems.

Most problems develop without clear causes, especially those caused by muscle imbalance. The questions below may help with further assessment of your foot problem.

Did the problem begin soon after a new activity?

Many people develop problems soon after they start an exercise program, change a current one, stop working out, change jobs, or change some other lifestyle habits. If a change in activity, for example, is associated with the onset of a foot problem, it may be that the activity is too much for your feet to handle. If it's your exercise program, you may be overtraining, which is a very common problem.

Did the problem begin soon after new or different shoes were worn?

Shoes are the cause of most foot problems, and this issue is discussed in detail in Section II: Shoes. If your foot problem begins soon after wearing a new or different pair of shoes, then the shoes may not match your foot properly. This could be related to an improper size, too much support, or other factors. Shoes that fit right are, at the very least, very comfortable.

Does the problem get better or worse with movement or rest?

If your foot problem feels better with movement, it's generally a good indication. As we move our muscles, they get warmed up and are able to function better. Sometimes an adequate warm up takes ten to fifteen minutes, and some problems may feel better only after this period of time. But don't push yourself if there's a lot of pain.

  If a problem worsens during activity, especially after you've had time to warm up, it usually means you should be resting to give the body a chance to heal. It may mean there's a more serious problem, but it could simply mean that the body needs more recovery time because of muscle inhibition. Pushing yourself in this situation often makes the problem worse and could lead to a chronic, recurring type of problem.

Is the problem better or worse at the end of the day?

Generally, if your problem feels worse at the end of the day, activity and/or weight bearing made it worse. In this case, it's the same consideration as in the question above–your foot may need more rest. In some cases, you may have accumulated fluid in your foot, ankle, and lower leg by the end of the day because your body is not able to circulate this fluid back through the veins. For example, it could be a circulatory problem, which is sometimes associated with a thyroid problem.

  Many people wear the wrong shoes, which can make an existing problem worse at the end of the day. But even when there is not a real problem to start with, your feet will be sore or "tired" after a day in bad shoes because they created a relatively minor problem throughout the day.

  If you feel better at the end of the day, it usually means activity has been helpful.

Is the problem better or worse in the morning?

After being off your feet all night, most mechanical problems will feel better in the morning because your foot had time to recover without mechanical stress. Certain problems may not follow this pattern. Plantar pain and the joint pain of arthritis may feel worse as soon as you start walking and gradually feel better after some movement. This may indicate a biochemical component to your problem (see Chapter 15), and it is often associated with too much calcium being deposited in the area during the night. A fracture may also feel worse at night and in the morning due to swelling.

Being off your feet can have effects similar to those of a good night's rest. If you feel better or worse after sitting for a while, the same factors may apply.

Are some of the toenails discolored or blackened?

This is usually indicative of shoes that don't fit properly. No matter what you're doing, the toenails should not become discolored if the shoe fits properly, barring trauma to the nail. This usually happens on the big toe, but any of the toes can be affected. In some cases, fungal infections cause blackened toenails.

Are there calluses in different places on both feet?

Slight callusing or thickening of the skin may be normal, especially if you spend time barefoot. But large calluses and ones that are painful are not normal. These are usually caused by muscle imbalance.

If you have calluses in different locations on both your feet, it may indicate significant muscle imbalance causing your feet to callus from uneven wear and tear. This imbalance may be in the foot, leg, or even the pelvis, causing one foot to move differently than the other. In addition, poor fitting shoes may aggravate the problem or even cause calluses to form, especially if one foot is larger than the other. Shoes should always fit the larger foot.

Are the wear patterns different on both shoes?

Like calluses, the wear pattern on your shoes can tell a story about foot balance. Shoe wear on the back of the heels, along the outside of the shoe, and near the ball of the foot should be similar in both shoes. If it's not, there may be muscle imbalance that's not allowing normal foot movement. As with calluses, this is usually caused by muscle imbalance, but the shoe itself can also be part of the problem.

Are footprints symmetrical?

Another clue that the feet are not balanced are your footprints. If you walk in the sand, dirt, or other area where you can see your footprints, they should show nearly identical patterns. The same is true for your shoe prints. Look for the prints to be facing slightly outward rather than straight. Prints that are facing straight forward or pointed outward too much may indicate a muscle imbalance in the pelvis, which affects how the feet hit the ground. If you use this assessment, be sure the ground is relatively flat, otherwise you will see a normal deviation in prints.

Does the problem area feel different or the same on the other foot?

If you have a problem area in your foot, feel all around the area. Then feel the same area on the other foot that has no pain. Both areas should normally feel about the same. While both sides of the body are not perfectly symmetrical, they are very similar. Many people become overly concerned about how a specific area looks or feels, when in fact, the other foot looks and feels the same, albeit without pain or disability. Since most problems are due to muscle imbalance, you will not see gross changes in the foot where there is discomfort. In some cases, swelling may be the only change, but sometimes even this is not detectable.

Are the symptoms the same in both feet?

Most foot problems occur on one side or the other, and rarely are there problems with identical patterns in both feet. When this does happen, it may simple muscle imbalance, but it could point to a more serious systemic condition, such as a spinal or circulatory problem or arthritis.

However, in many situations, general foot discomfort at the end of the day is simply due to wearing shoes not meant for your feet. This becomes obvious when you take your shoes off and move around a bit, only to find significant relief.

PROBLEM AREAS

Foot and ankle problems are a true epidemic, with certain areas most vulnerable. Men, women, and children can develop a variety of problems, including first metatarsal jam, sprained ankle, plantar pain, and a variety of other fore-, mid-, and hindfoot problems.

First Metatarsal Jam

Excess pressure and stress through the big toe into the first metatarsal joint is a very common problem. It's almost always due to wearing shoes that are too small. In rare cases, it is due to the person kicking hard objects with the front of the foot. This is sometimes seen in construction workers or carpenters who may use their feet as a tool without effective work boots. In some athletes, such as cyclists, football players, or baseball players, the same injury frequently occurs due to tight shoes or to kicking a ball, being hit by a ball, or jamming a foot into the ground.

This injury involves the bone of the big toe, the phalanx, jamming back into the first metatarsal bone (see Figure 4.2). The first metatarsal joint, between the two bones, becomes inflamed and painful. In some situations, when the onset of the problem is very slow, the joint does not elicit pain, but rather the foot adapts by adjusting to the problem by creating another problem elsewhere that is secondary to the first metatarsal. In a real sense, other parts of the foot are sacrificed to take away some of the stress of the first metatarsal. This is not an uncommon way for the body to adapt when a very important structure, such as the first metatarsal joint, has excessive stress placed upon it. Many ankle, heel, knee, and other problems may be due to a first metatarsal jam.

This first metatarsal jam can be assessed using two key indicators: the toe itself and the shoe. In the toe, pain and swelling in the area of the first metatarsal joint is common. Even a relatively minor jamming of the metatarsal joint over a long period will cause swelling of the joint. This is evident by a slight enlargement of the joint, with a warm feeling to touch due to inflammation.

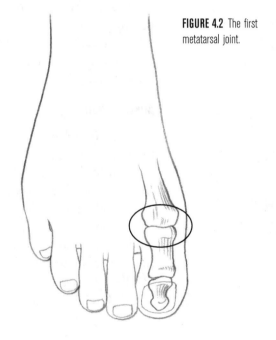

FIGURE 4.2 The first metatarsal joint.

Sometimes a discolored toenail–the result of constant pressure from a shoe that's too tight–is obvious. This is especially common in people who wear tight shoes and are very active, such as athletes. Even a single long workout or race in shoes that don't fit properly could create a first metatarsal problem complete with blackened toenail. The reason for the toenail's discoloration is tiny hemorrhages underneath the nail, just like other bruises.

The shoes can also give clues to a first metatarsal jam. Because the foot is wedged forward into the shoe, many toenails can jam into the front of the shoe. Over time, the toenail can bore a hole into the shoe, but more often shoes are discarded before this happens. Even a toenail that is not very long can do this if the shoe is sufficiently tight. This wear pattern can usually be felt inside the shoe. With your fingers, feel inside the shoe in the area where your toenail would rub. You may feel a roughened spot and in some cases, a layer of material may have worn off the inside of the shoe. Specifically, this means the shoe is too short.

Keeping the toenails properly trimmed can be helpful, but wearing the proper shoe size is necessary to prevent a recurrence of the problem.

Assessing the shoe further can be helpful. If you have a removable insole, take it out and study it. Look at the wear pattern, especially the indentation made from the toes. Observe the areas compressed by the toes that are not completely on the insert, like they should be. Toes that overlap the top of the insert obviously indicate a too-small shoe.

In a foot that has an atypical shape, or in people with unusual circumstances, such as a job-related pounding or sports that require kicking, other metatarsals can have the same fate. In addition, other traumas can create this problem as well, such as falling while wearing soft shoes or severely stubbing your toe.

Turf toe is a similar condition, where the toe is injured during forced metatarsal movements, such as a push-off injury or other trauma. It usually includes the sesamoid bones under the first metatarsal joint, which may become inflamed and sometimes fractured. This is evident from local tenderness or pain on the bottom of the foot under the first metatarsal joint.

ANKLE SPRAIN

As mentioned previously, every day in the United States more than twenty-five thousand people sprain an ankle. In most cases, the outside portion of the foot and ankle are affected, with symptoms of pain being the most common complaint. Swelling is the most common sign. Most people who sprain their ankle don't do serious damage. However, about half of those with a previous history of this problem will sprain their ankle again due to incomplete healing causing muscle imbalance, with the peroneal muscles being the most common to become inhibited. Studies show that people who wear shoes with air cells in the heel are more than four times more likely to sprain an ankle, and those who wear "high-top" athletic shoes may actually have a higher incidence of ankle sprains than do those who wear regular athletic shoes.

The typical ankle sprain is associated with injuries of ligaments, muscles, and tendons on the outside of the ankle. This injury is sometimes serious. Although only about 10 percent of those who sprain their ankle will fracture a bone, the most important concern following an ankle sprain is making sure there is no fracture.

Some experts suggest everyone who sprains an ankle have an X ray, the only way to determine if a fracture is present. But others say this leads to many unnecessary X rays. One issue is clear: Every person with a sprained ankle should be treated as an individual. A professional consensus, known as the "Ottawa Ankle Rules," uses specific questions and examination of key areas to help doctors determine the risk of bone fracture.

After spraining your ankle, a question that should be asked is whether you can bear weight on that foot and ankle, even if it's painful. A second question is whether you can walk four steps, unaided, even with pain or a limp right after your injury. A health professional may also ask you to do this if you go to the emergency room. If you're able to accomplish these tasks, an X ray may not be recommended because the chances of a fracture are extremely low.

However, despite your ability to bear weight or walk, certain pain areas may still indicate a potential fracture leading a doctor to X-ray your ankle. If there is pain in either bone of the inner or outer ankle, or pain or tenderness at the base of the fifth metatarsal, or the navicular bone, the risk of fracture is higher.

PLANTAR PAIN

Pain in the bottom of the foot, generally referred to as plantar pain, can come from a variety of sources. Almost all plantar pain is functional, and therefore the problem can usually be corrected conservatively. If you have plantar pain, first carefully check the skin since a small cut, splinter, piece of glass, wart, or other similar problem can be the cause.

Plantar pain inside the foot, especially in the mid- or hindfoot, frequently comes from tight plantar muscles. This tightness is most often secondary to other muscle inhibition. A "diagnosis" of *plantar fasciitis* is not indicative of the cause of the problem, and no single remedy for this named condition has proven successful. Two people with the same plantar pain due to tight plantar muscles may have very different causes.

A so-called bone "spur" may be present in some chronic cases of plantar pain associated with long-term plantar muscle tightness. In this case, the tendon of the plantar muscles that attaches to the calcaneus (heel) bone may contain high levels of calcium, known as *calcium deposits*. On an X ray, this gives the appearance of a pointed "spur," which can give a false impression of a pointed sharp object in your foot. This is another example of the body compensating for a problem: To further strengthen the area, the body deposits calcium in the tendon. In addition to local treatment, chronic problems such as this may require improvements to the body chemistry (see Chapter 15).

Other problems are much less common causes of plantar pain. A *neuroma* (discussed below) can cause forefoot plantar pain. A hidden *stress fracture* is also possible, which may or may not be found on an X ray. *Tarsal tunnel syndrome* produces diffuse symptoms over the bottom of the foot. The cause is often instability of the calcaneus bone from muscle imbalance and/or trauma. Chronic tarsal tunnel syndrome can result in numbness or tingling in the bottom of the foot. Arthritis is also a possible cause of plantar pain, but in most cases a diagnosis of arthritis has already been made.

LIFESTYLE FOOT DEFORMITIES

True foot deformities are relatively rare; but deformities due to foot abuse are common. Wearing improper shoes can cause these lifestyle foot deformities. Forefoot deformities are especially common in women, who experience them nine times more often than men. Prevention is relatively simple, but once deformities develop they can't be reversed.

In the forefoot, two of the most common deformities are *bunions* (hallux valgus) and *hammertoes*. Bunions are very common in women because of the types of shoes many women wear—too narrow and too short. A bunion is an enlargement of the bone (the first metatarsal) and joint at the ball of the foot. The problem has a slow onset, taking years to develop. The changes are permanent, with pain and swelling the most common complaint. A similar problem can occur on the outside of the foot with the fifth toe, and this condition is termed a *bunionette*.

Hammertoes are common lifestyle deformities of one or more of the four smaller toes. This is usually the result of wearing tight-fitting shoes for many years. Occasionally hammertoes can be the result of trauma, such as a severe injury or fracture. Hammertoes are a deformity of the second joint, while *claw toes* are a similar deformity of the first joint.

Conservative therapy for mild and moderate bunions, hammertoes, and claw toes involves wearing shoes that fit properly, are usually wider in the toe area, and do not have heels, which shift weight onto the forefoot. Balancing the foot muscles if there is a problem can be very helpful to reduce pain, but proper shoe wear must be maintained. For those who get no relief from conservative care or for those who are unwilling to wear proper shoes, surgery is the last resort to relieve pain and dysfunction.

NEUROMAS

A neuroma in the foot is called an *interdigital neuroma,* or *Morton's neuroma,* and is technically not a true neuroma. It is caused by a thickening of the small nerve as it enters the toes, usually occurring between the third and fourth toes (occasionally between the second and third toes, and very rarely in the other toe areas). Neuromas are five times more common in women who wear tight shoes.

Interdigital neuromas cause burning pain in the bottom of the forefoot. They are usually aggravated by activity and feel better with rest. Pain can be elicited by pushing up on the toes from the bottom of the foot while squeezing the toes together; this is a common test for neuromas because X rays don't show their presence.

Conservative therapy for neuromas begins with properly fitting shoes that are usually wider in the toe area and have no heels. Balancing the muscles that influence the feet can be very helpful for symptomatic relief, but proper shoe fit must be maintained. In severe cases, a steroid injection may reduce the need for surgery by 50 percent. Surgical removal is a last resort.

INGROWN TOENAIL

An ingrown toenail is a common foot problem. It usually occurs in the big toe because of poor fitting shoes, improper nail trimming, or both. The area becomes inflamed and painful and can lead to secondary fungal or bacterial infections.

Conservative treatment is usually effective, and this includes accommodative shoes. Warm foot soaks and proper nail trimming are also very effective. Trimming the nail is best accomplished by cutting it straight across rather than on a curve.

STRESS FRACTURES

In addition to fractured bones due to trauma, *stress fractures* are not uncommon in the foot and ankle. Stress fractures are usually less severe but they can be significant problems, and they typically occur from repetitive overuse or a sudden increase in activity, which the person is not used to. In some cases, metabolic causes are evident, such as with amenorrhea (the lost of menstrual period) in women or osteoporosis in either sex. In these cases, there may be more than one stress fracture.

In addition to the leg bones (tibia and fibula), common sites of stress fractures in the foot include the metatarsal bones and navicular bone.

Pain from a stress fracture typically improves with rest and worsens with activity. There is often some swelling in the area, but sometimes it's not noticeable. The swelling around the bone may prevent a proper diagnosis by X ray within the first two weeks of injury. Only after some healing has taken place will the X ray show the problem. In these situations, a bone scan may locate the stress fracture.

In a healthy person, most stress fractures will heal well without major therapy. Rest, cooling the site of the fracture, cessation of weight-bearing exercise, and hard-soled flat shoes are often sufficient, but each case must be treated individually. Aspirin and other NSAIDs (non-steroidal anti-inflammatory drugs) must be *avoided* as they can delay bone healing. See Chapter 13 for information about using acupressure to control pain.

THERAPEUTIC OPTIONS

Once you have assessed your feet, you will have a better idea of the nature of your foot problem and will be better able to decide your next step. You have three options: leave things alone and let your body recover, help your body with some conservative remedies, or seek professional help. In some situations, you may need to try two or all three of these options before you find the correct remedy.

HEAL THYSELF

Often a foot problem is self-limiting, meaning the body will correct the problem without any other help. If you're allowing your body to fix your feet, give the process some time. However, if the problem is not beginning to improve in a reasonable period, more help may be needed. An acute foot problem, one involving trauma, for example, that does not start to feel better within twenty-four to forty-eight hours may require some assistance. For more chronic problems, such as the nontraumatic type, one or two weeks should be sufficient time for at least some improvement to be seen.

In allowing your body to fix itself, rest may be the key. One of the most powerful of therapies, rest can be a double-edged sword if overused. The key with rest is knowing when and when not to use it.

Many active people often have trouble resting when they should. Rest is the best way for the body to recover. This recovery may be from a day at work, a long day of hiking, or some hard exercise. Recovery is essential for the body to build up the muscles, allowing them to get stronger or more functional. Without recovery there could be some form of injury that might not exhibit any symptoms until the problem gets worse.

Too much rest can also be a problem. The most common example is inactivity: Some people rest all the time. Sometimes we use a minor problem as an excuse to rest, when in fact the reason for the minor problem may be inactivity itself.

ASSISTED HEALING

A variety of self-administered remedies can be used for many foot problems. But if the time comes, finding a health professional can be very important. Both subjects are addressed in later chapters. Fortunately, the majority of foot problems are not serious. However, almost all foot problems are accompanied by pain, the topic of our next chapter.

5

FOOT PAIN

Virtually all serious foot problems are associated with some type of pain. This chapter defines pain in its different forms and discusses common pain patterns in the foot associated with specific foot problems.

WHAT IS PAIN?

Pain is a sensation our body uses to influence our judgment. When our foot gives us pain, we usually don't use it the same way or we rest it. Pain tells us something is not right–this is the most important aspect of pain. Ignoring it can lead to more serious problems. Resisting pain, such as when we try masking it with painkillers, can make things worse. The earliest symptoms of pain should be heeded. The sooner you address a painful foot, the quicker the problem can be resolved either by your body itself, by self remedy, or with the help of a professional.

Pain can be likened to one of the senses as it is mediated through the body by special nerve fibers and registered in the brain as pain. Technically, however, pain is not a sense like our sense of taste or smell, but an emotion. If you have pain in your foot, the nerve endings for pain (called *nociceptors*) have detected a problem and sent a message to your brain's emotional center, where pain is experienced.

Pain is usually triggered by damage to some body part such as a ligament, tendon, muscle, bone, or skin. In some cases, just the *perception* of pain is sufficient to trigger pain.

THREE TYPES OF PAIN

Pain can originate from one, two, or three different types of stimulation or stress:

1. *Mechanical stress* can trigger pain from trauma or swelling. This includes physical trauma such as a sprained ankle, a jammed toe, or pressure from swelling. Tight shoes are common sources of mechanical pain.
2. *Chemical stress* may produce pain through the chemical stimulation of nerve endings. The chemical by-products of both inflammation (including histamine) and muscle fatigue (such as lactic acid) are responsible for chemical pain.
3. Thermal stress is associated with pain from temperature extremes. Heat or cold can produce pain through the stimulation of nerve endings. In some situations, cold pain may begin below 59°F and heat pain at or above 113°F.

It is not unusual to develop pain from more than one source. For example, mechanical stress on a tightened muscle and the chemical stress that results through the accumulation of metabolic by-products such as lactic acid can both cause the pain accompanying a muscle cramp. And the mechanical stresses of both trauma and swelling as well as the chemical stress of inflammation can produce pain in an ankle sprain.

PAIN QUALITY

The quality of pain may be associated with its source. Although most people may complain just of pain, this complaint is usually too general for assessment purposes. If we can be more specific in describing our pain, it may give us more of a clue about the type and source of the pain, which may help us remedy it.

For example, mechanical pain is associated with descriptions such as *stabbing* or *knifelike pressure* or *grabbing*. If the mechanical pain is around blood vessels (specifically, an artery), the words *pulsating, throbbing,* or *pounding* are often used. In this case the problem would be deeper in the foot, where the arteries are located, rather than closer to the surface.

Chemical pain can be described as being *hot, searing,* or *burning*. In these cases there is usually a need to consider the body chemistry along with mechanical causes of the problem. Inflammation is commonly associated with this type of pain. The remedy may have to include diet or nutritional changes to completely solve the problem, as discussed in Chapter 15.

Pain is also unlike our senses in that you become more sensitive to the pain as it becomes more chronic. Over time, chronic pain will generally become increasingly more evident and you may be more aware of it. Our senses of taste, smell, touch, etc., do just the opposite with long-term stimulation—our brain becomes *less* aware of the sensation after long-term constant stimulation.

Some individuals are more tolerant of pain than others. The reason is probably the natural pain-control mechanisms within nervous system. Two important chemicals (called neurotransmitters), serotonin and enkephalin, regulate this pain control. These chemicals act to diminish pain in the spinal cord. In addition, other naturally occurring chemicals called *endorphins* in the brain have opiate-like qualities and play a part in pain control.

Pain control techniques are discussed in Chapter 14, but simple, light stimulation on the skin may help reduce pain. This is accomplished by rubbing the skin at or near an area of pain. When people are injured, they typically, and usually subconsciously, rub the area of injury as a way to control pain. This action stimulates certain areas in the nervous system to block some pain and is the same mechanism as employed by *transcutaneous electrical nerve stimulation devices,* which are used in patients with extreme or continual pain. It may also be the same mechanism that makes acupuncture successful in pain control.

FOOT PAIN DIAGRAM

Some serious foot problems show specific areas of pain. These are highlighted in Figures 5.1a and 5.1b.

On the bottom of the foot (Figure 5.1a), some common plantar pain locations include the following:

- first metatarsal joint pain
- sesamoid bone pain
- plantar wart pain
- other metatarsal pain
- two common areas of plantar muscle tightness

On the top and side of the foot (Figure 5.1b), some common pain locations include the following:

- bunion pain
- common locations of hammertoe, claw toe, and corn pain
- ingrown toenail pain

- bunionette pain
- midfoot fracture pain

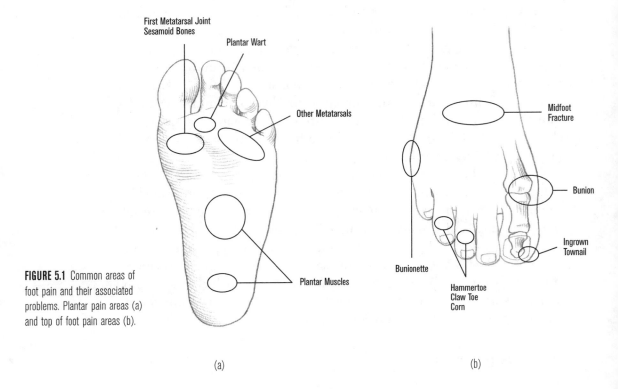

FIGURE 5.1 Common areas of foot pain and their associated problems. Plantar pain areas (a) and top of foot pain areas (b).

(a)   (b)

Most foot and ankle pain will improve with rest, i.e., by being off your feet, especially following a night's rest. Pain during the night may indicate a more serious problem such as an infection.

Perhaps the most common cause of any pain in the foot is the types of shoes that are worn. This is the subject of the next section.

SECTION TWO

S H O E S

Nothing influences the foot as much as shoes. Nothing does the foot as much potential harm as shoes. And nothing restores normal function as quickly as when shoes are removed. However, in many situations, shoes are a necessity for foot protection.

The main purpose of shoes is to protect the feet from potentially dangerous objects or rough surfaces, and at times to protect against the cold. Any purpose beyond these functions is strictly for costume. In very rare instances, people with particular foot problems may need special shoes, such as those with birth deformities or those who have seriously damaged their feet through accidents or other similar instances. These issues are not discussed in this book.

This section includes a brief history of shoes, including their use for function and costume, and how they are made. It details how shoes can harm the feet and how to avoid such situations, including how to find the shoes that best fit your feet. Discussions on orthotics and other foot supports are included.

6

A BRIEF HISTORY OF SHOES AND MANUFACTURING

For millions of years, the human foot has been either bare or covered with very simple footwear to protect the bottoms of the feet. Sandals were the common covering in warmer climates, with moccasins used in colder environments for added warmth. These sparse foot coverings were and are adequate to protect the bottom of the foot from sharp rocks and rough terrain. Foot problems due to being barefoot consisted of the occasional laceration or deep thorn. Today, simple sandals and moccasins are still the most common footwear worldwide.

With the advent of today's modern shoes came a whole array of foot problems complete with companies that made therapeutic devices and professionals to treat such conditions. Many companies and individuals have benefited, as the shoe industry and those products and services connected with the epidemic of foot problems are big business. Larger shoe companies such as Nike generate annual revenues of more than $10 billion, with those of smaller companies like Reebok around $3 billion.

HISTORY

From the earliest times, shoes were made with an important function in mind: to protect the bottoms of the feet. But as society evolved, shoes found their place in costume and ceremony. In these situations, special shoes were made very fancy and with lavish design, but they were used only occasionally. Because of their infrequent use, comfort and function were not an important focus. Today we've adapted that same attitude, but there is tremendous competition on a daily basis to wear the most fancy of shoes, no price barred.

In the Middle Ages, a peaked shoe called the Crackow became popular. This had a toe so long that walking was extremely difficult. It was also dangerous, not only for the person wearing it but also for those nearby, and eventually the passage of laws prohibited their use. The Duckbill shoe followed, and again laws were enacted limiting its maximum width to 5 1/2 inches.

For most of humanity, shoes were made straight with left and right being identical. Records show that from the fourteenth century B.C. in Egypt until the mid 1800s, shoes were essentially produced the same way by the trade—by lapstone and hammer. For centuries, shoemakers kept secret the measurements of their client's feet to help ensure continued business. Today, a similar approach is evident, as one size does not fit all feet the same.

In 1845 the Rolling machine, followed by the invention of the sewing machine a year later, dramatically changed the shoe industry. By 1860 other more effective machines were developed for shoemaking. The next manufacturing breakthrough came in 1875, when Charles Goodyear, Jr. developed a new machine that made shoes using a new material called rubber, a substance invented by his father.

Today most shoes are made on machines, but they also require manual assembly. The manufacturing of many shoes, especially sneakers and so-called sport or athletic shoes produced by big companies, takes place in third world countries because it's very cheap to make them there, often a dollar per pair or less.

The problems caused by today's shoes are not unlike those experienced during the Elizabethan times. Modern shoes are made for style (costume) first, with comfort taking a back seat in many cases and function usually not even considered (the differences between real and perceived shoe function is discussed in the next chapter). Interestingly, today's fancy shoes are also shown to cause health problems, and some medical experts have called for warnings about their dangers. A 1997 *British Journal of Sports Medicine* paper by Steven Robbins, Ph.D., described the hazards of deceptive advertising of athletic footwear. Speaking about modern athletic shoes, Robbins states, "deceptive advertising of protective devices [in shoes] may represent a public health hazard and may have to be eliminated presumably through regulation." Others have called for Public Health awareness. Whether this leads to warning labels is yet to be determined.

SHOE STRUCTURE

With seemingly endless styles of shoes, they all have a very similar basic structure with two parts: a *lower* and an *upper*. Following is an example of the general structure of many common shoes starting from the ground up. Many shoe parts have more than one name, and many shoes don't contain all parts. A basic shoe is depicted in Figure 6.1.

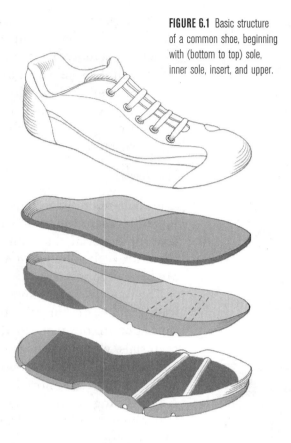

FIGURE 6.1 Basic structure of a common shoe, beginning with (bottom to top) sole, inner sole, insert, and upper.

THE LOWER

The *sole* (from the Latin word *solea*, meaning soil or ground) is our contact with the ground. The *outer sole* is the material that is in direct contact with the ground. This material can be made of rubber, leather, or synthetic materials, and sometimes a combination of materials is used. Soles come in a wide range of thickness and flexibility. The sole should be made to provide traction and resist slipping.

The *innersole* (or midsole) is attached to the top part of the outer sole. It helps in the attachment of upper to lower and provides additional cushioning. Many shoes have insoles that are treated with chemicals to prevent bacterial growth.

Some shoes contain another layer on top of the sole called an *insert* that is said to provide more support by attempting to hold up parts of the foot. It certainly adds more cushioning, but also takes up more room in the shoe. Inserts are usually made of various synthetic fabrics, soft and hard, and sometimes leather, which is perhaps the best material to use. An *orthotic* is a type of insert. These are discussed in Chapter 9.

Most shoes are manufactured using a *last*–a general model of a foot. The term comes from Old English, *laest,* which means barefoot. Lasts were originally carved out of wood, but today they are plastic or metal. They are made for manufacturing purposes. Lasts provide a working structure by which the shoe is made. Manufacturers say there are two kinds of feet, and therefore two general forms of lasts exist, a *straight* and *curved* last. *Straight lasted* shoes are straighter in appearance, and *curve lasted* shoes more curved overall.

The upper part of the shoe attaches to the last two different ways. A *slip lasted* shoe has the upper part wrapped around the lower sole and glued and is more like a sock. It is usually softer and more flexible, especially in the sole. The more traditional shoe style, especially for dress shoes, is *board lasted*, which is stapled, tacked, or sometimes glued to the sole. A board-lasted shoe is more rigid, especially the sole. Some shoes are slip lasted in the front and board lasted in the back, with other variations used in manufacturing today.

THE UPPER

The remainder of the shoe above the innersole and insert is called the *upper*. Its main function is to hold the lower onto the foot. A *welt* is a strip of material that joins the upper to the lower. The majority of shoes are welted by Goodyear-welt construction, although some welts are only decorative.

The most functional material for an upper is leather. It not only allows the foot to "breath" by allowing hot air around the foot to escape, but it conforms to the size and shape of the foot. Synthetic materials, which resist water better, do not conform to the foot well and remain ill fitted unless the shoes fit perfectly from the beginning. Cotton uppers are more benign, as long as the fit is relatively good.

Depending on the shoe style, the upper can include many other parts, including *laces* and a *tongue*, which protects the top of the foot. The *counter* is the heel area and may include a *stiffener* for added support. The *collar* is a soft, thicker ring around the shoe opening common in sports shoes, as are *linings*, which provide added comfort. *Shanks* are used for added support when there is a heel, raising the back of the foot higher than the front. It's usually made from metal, plastic, or wood and supports the space on the bottom of the shoe between the heel and toes, keeping it from collapsing.

SHOE STYLES

There are generally considered to be eight different shoe styles. These are listed below. Some shoes today represent a combination of styles.

1. *Boots.* These are shoes that extend above the ankle. They can be casual or dressy.
2. *Clogs.* These are made with a thick wooden or cork sole and have no back. They probably originated in rural Europe in the 1300s. They can be casual or dressy.

3. *Lace-ups.* These traditional shoes, such as the Oxford, are for casual, dress, and formal wear. They use laces for a better fit. Many sports shoes are considered lace-ups.
4. *Moccasins.* These are perhaps the first shoes ever made, along with sandals. The name is from the Algonquians of North America. *Imitation moccasins* originated in Norway and are popular today as *loafers*. They are usually casual, but some are dressy.
5. *Monks.* These are similar to lace-ups but instead of lacing have a strap that comes over the top of the shoe to adjust the fit. They can be used for casual or dress shoes. Some sports shoes are made with this style.
6. *Mules.* These are backless shoes, with or without heels. The flat soft versions are *slippers*. They can be for very casual to very formal wear.
7. *Pumps.* These are the traditional, elegant, high-heeled shoes with open front tops or toe boxes, often with long spiked heels. These are usually for dress or formal wear.
8. *Sandals.* Some have heels, others are flat, and some are thongs, while others have fancy lacing up the leg. Wooden sandals (*geta*) are of Japanese origin. Sandals can be casual or dressy.

Although times have changed we can see from history that much is still the same. We can make more shoes with modern machinery and synthetic materials, but despite our understanding of biomechanics, shoes still influence the foot more than any other single factor, and probably all other factors combined. More importantly, shoes are the cause of most foot problems. Just how this happens is discussed in the next chapter.

7

HOW SHOES CAN HARM

When was the very first time the human foot was injured by a shoe? Probably the first time it was worn. Nothing is more stable, supportive, shock protective, and efficient than bare feet. As soon as a shoe is placed on the foot, there is a loss of stability and the potential for injury. Perhaps the very first shoe-related injury was a twisted ankle due to the surprised instability. Or worse, being overtaken by a wild tiger due to slower running speed or poor maneuverability in shoes. Though most of us don't have to run from wild animals, our shoes can still be dangerous.

Perhaps the first published scientific evidence describing the harm caused by shoes came in 1954, when researchers Basmajian and Bentzon measured the electrical activity in foot muscles using an electromyographic device. This study showed that when shoes were placed on the feet, certain muscles lost significant function.

Since that time, many other studies have been published in medical journals showing the dangers associated with shoes. Some of these are listed in the bibliography in the back of this book.

There are a variety of specific problems associated with wearing shoes. I've broken these subjects down to four general categories: weight bearing, foot-sense and orientation, muscle and bone support, and gait.

WEIGHT BEARING

Our feet support our entire body's weight. Normally, this weight is distributed through specific areas of the feet in order to bear weight most efficiently. Efficient weight-bearing distribution reduces the risk of injury. When we wear shoes, our weight distribution can change, often with more weight going through a smaller area of the foot. An extreme example of this is wearing high-heeled shoes, especially those with very small pointed heels and a small toe box. In this case, all the body's weight is directed into the ground through a very small area—through the heel and the front of the foot. When we wear a flat shoe or are barefoot, the distribution of weight is over a larger area, although even a flat shoe can interfere with our weight bearing.

This example is easily seen with the following experiment. Place your dampened feet on a flat, dry paper towel and stand up. Step off the towel and observe your footprints. Drawing an outline around the print may help you see it better. Next, take a pair of flat shoes that you have worn for a while and observe the area of wear—this will be mostly the back outer corner of your heel and the ball of the foot, and sometimes along the outer edge of the shoe. Now compare the size of your footprint with the area of wear pattern on your shoes. In most cases, your footprint area will be larger, sometimes a lot larger. In other words, your contact with the ground is greater when barefoot than when wearing shoes.

The surface area that makes contact with the ground is a significant factor associated with many types of foot problems. For example, if the weight of your body is forced through a smaller area of your foot (i.e., less surface area), more stress is induced in your foot. Instead, your foot is supposed to disperse the weight-bearing stress through a *greater* surface area. In addition, with less surface area making contact with the ground, the body has a lessened ability to maintain proper overall balance.

The flatter and thinner the sole of your shoe, the more your weight bearing is likely to be more natural—like a barefoot state. Changing to this type of shoe could have significant benefits for your feet, but as discussed in the next chapter, you must do this carefully if you're used to shoes with thick shoes, high heels, or a lot of support.

IMPACT

Our weight-bearing contact with the ground is closely associated with the foot's *impact* with the ground. Impact is intimately connected to foot-sense.

For many years, sport-shoe manufacturers focused on impact, promoting shoes with so-called shock absorbing materials to protect us from the impact forces that supposedly caused injury. But after decades of scientific research, experts are unable to demonstrate that our feet are vulnerable to injury from the result of impact, whether from standing, walking, running, or jumping. In fact, what the studies show is that there is no difference in injury rates between running on hard surfaces and soft surfaces or between runners who have high or low impact with the ground.

Certainly, *excessive* impact will injure our feet. However, the action of standing, walking, running, and performing other common types of physical activity is quite natural—our feet are made for these activities and the normal impacts associated with them. The forces of impact are a natural phenomenon our feet are made to deal with. Actually, our feet utilize the impact with the ground to decide how much muscle work is needed to stand, walk, or run most efficiently. This action is mediated through the nerves and muscles in the feet.

The muscle response to impact also affects comfort. For this reason, all shoes, from the moment you put on a new pair to those that appear too old and worn out, should be completely comfortable (this is discussed in Chapter 8). Otherwise, the shoe should not be worn because of the risk of foot damage.

Still other benefits are obtained from our constant impact with the ground. Bone strength can be improved in those who perform activities that result in harder impact, such as jogging or running, especially when compared to activities that have low or almost no impact such as swimming. Therefore, if some shoes really had the capability to reduce shock or impact, it would clearly harm the foot, with each and every step.

The effect of normal impact on cartilage may also be benign. However, studies show that extremely high impacts may be a problem, but these are not the same intensities experienced by runners, for example, who have perhaps the highest impact of all the common activities. Animal studies demonstrate damage from high impact; however, animals don't normally experience high impact either.

Human studies have long shown that our highest natural impact activity, running, does not cause osteoarthritis—a type of arthritis caused by physical and chemical stress that damages cartilage around the joints.

SHOCK ABSORPTION

Shock absorption is another common phrase promoted by sport-shoe and other companies. The remedy for the notion that shock and impact is dangerous has led to the idea that we must cushion our feet, especially when walking, jogging, running, or performing other physical activity. But because a material has good shock-absorbing ability, it does not mean it can accomplish this inside a shoe. In fact, shoe materials with good shock-absorbency properties are not effective enough to reduce stress in the foot during physical activity. This is because shock absorption in the feet occurs at the same level of intensity whether we wear shoes or not.

Cushioning is a concept most people relate to comfort and safety. Cushioning can protect your feet against bruising if you should step on a hard object like a sharp stone. However, cushioning can have drawbacks. Shoes that are too cushioned can give the nervous system the improper perception that the impact is much less than it actually is, which can result in the inadequate or improper response by the foot (and rest of the body) to the actual impact. In the course of a walk, run, or all day moving about in your shoes, this could add up to be a significant cause of injury.

Cushioning is more common in the popular, expensive sports shoes. In a December 1997 issue of the *British Journal of Sports Medicine*, researchers Robbins and Waked state, "Expensive athletic shoes are deceptively advertised to safeguard well through 'cushioning impact' yet account for 123% greater injury frequency than the cheapest ones."

Remember, regardless of the shock absorbing devices in the shoe or level of cushioning, shock absorption in the foot is the same. This is one reason why shock-absorbing and impact-cushioning materials used in many sports shoes account for a 123 percent greater injury frequency in comparison to plain, unsupported inexpensive shoes.

If we see the impact force of being on our feet as a way for the body to naturally adapt to the impact, it's easier to understand how shoes can interfere with our natural mechanisms.

SUPPORT

Many shoes have a so-called "support system" built into them. This may be a simple insert or a complex arrangement of built-up stabilizing structures with fancy names. Most of these exist for marketing reasons and provide no real function, as discussed in Chapter 9.

Normally, the body reacts to influences placed on it, and the feet are a good example. For the vast majority of people, the feet are most supported when bare. Put on a shoe and we can lose some natural muscle support. If the shoe has a lot of supports built-in, we may lose even more natural support from our feet. This is because our feet give way to the external support. In a real sense, our feet have no reason to support themselves as much if something is doing the job for them. The same is true for any action taken to interfere and replace the body's natural function. Bed rest is a more obvious example. Potential side effects from bed rest include muscle atrophy (up to 1.5 percent of muscle mass lost per day), reduced aerobic conditioning (about 1.5 percent lost per day), significant bone mineral loss, and risk of blood clots. So if bed rest is ordered, it must be for a very important reason.

Likewise, if we need added support for our feet because we have a se-rious problem, it may be helpful. But support the feet when they don't truly need it and you're asking for trouble. For most people, this need may not exist. Some people, however, may need extra support because they have stayed in shoes with too much support for too long, thereby weakening the natural support mechanisms—the muscles. For these in-dividuals, their feet don't feel right without the added support. Wean-ing off oversupported shoes and strengthening the muscles of the feet can break this vicious cycle; both these topics are discussed in Section III: Treatment.

Support systems in many shoes contribute to a thicker heel area. When barefoot, our heel and forefoot are at about the same level, but most shoes are made so that our heel is higher than the rest of our foot. This unnatural state can ultimately result in reduced muscle function in the gastrocnemius and soleus and in the tibialis anterior. When jog-ging or running, this situation may change, as discussed below.

FOOT-SENSE AND ORIENTATION

Don't overlook the importance of foot-sense. Within the foot are im-portant nerve endings that sense foot contact with the ground. This in-formation is sent to the brain and spinal cord so we can respond appropriately to activities of the feet and help regulate all movement and body position. In effect, we orient ourselves—our whole body—as a result of foot-sense.

The primary reason for many common foot injuries is the *lack of feedback* from the foot *despite the same level of shock absorption*. This can be the result of increased thickness of the sole or the synthetic ma-terials used in many shoes. In other words, the soles of our feet are not able to properly communicate with the ground.

The relationship between reduced foot-sense and its contribution to injury has been understood in scientific circles for almost forty years.

K-SENSE

Because we are less able to communicate with the ground when we wear shoes, our feet are less able to adapt to the normal impact of reg-ular activity. And it's not just our feet, but our whole body. The result is a loss of *kinesthetic sense,* or k-sense, meaning our nervous system is less aware of our foot position, and therefore corresponding body po-sition, than it should be. Our body cannot adapt properly to normal walking, running, or virtually any movement. K-sense provides us with specific information about our movements, changes in posture, and the mechanical stress on muscles and joints. A loss of k-sense also can have an adverse effect on our orientation.

An example of k-sense can help us understand how important it can be. Getting through an obstacle course requires great k-sense. But everyday activity can be an obstacle course for our feet. If we're walking through a crowded restaurant dinning room to get to our table, we may have to squeeze past chairs, people, other tables, and perhaps even a wet floor to avoid running into these obstructions. We rely on our natural k-sense to do this.

It's been known for a long time that k-sense is reduced in the elderly and is the reason why walking through a restaurant may be more difficult or dangerous for them. But recently, it's been shown that even young people who have worn thick-soled shoes can also have significantly reduced k-sense.

Reduced k-sense can lead to injury at any age. But in the elderly, this problem can increase the incidence of falls that result in hip fractures, which are very serious. Hip fractures usually begin a rapid decline in overall health, with many patients dying within one year.

MUSCLE AND BONE SUPPORT

Muscles move bones, and if the muscles are not functioning properly, the bones move incorrectly and do not maintain proper foot posture. This can also adversely influence the joints and ligaments.

Perhaps the best indication that foot muscles are functioning properly while in a shoe—and therefore that the shoe matches the foot well—is comfort. If, at the end of the day, your feet are "tired" and sore, it's probably due to muscle dysfunction caused by your shoes. When trying on new shoes, use comfort to help you decide that the shoe is not interfering with muscle function. Shoes, inserts, orthotics, heel supports, or items that are not completely comfortable or make your shoe too small don't match the needs of your feet and may cause muscle imbalance.

However, comfort can be misleading. As discussed above, you may be "addicted" to oversupported shoes and not feel right in any other type of shoe, despite the problems being created. It's not until the problem becomes symptomatic that the problems are evident.

Most foot problems are associated with poor muscle function. Poor muscle function infers imbalance, which usually causes the bones to attain a poor postural position. The notion that a particular support can keep the bones of the foot in proper alignment is very misleading and an opinion not supported by scientific research.

GAIT

Balance is an important component of normal movement or normal gait. When balance is disturbed due to improper shoes, muscle imbalance and irregular gait follow. At best, the body will compensate for muscle imbalance with significantly more muscle activity. This can cause the body to use much more energy than normal to accomplish the same movement. In other words, an irregular gait wastes energy.

An irregular gait can also lead to an injury not only in the foot, but in the knee, pelvis, low back, or some other areas. Even the shoulders, neck, and head can be affected. Because of the importance of the hip joint during movement, the hips are particularly vulnerable to injury when there is a gait problem.

Abnormal changes in gait are common in the elderly. These are sometimes attributed to the so-called natural aging process in the feet—the loss of elasticity and arch function resulting in reduced foot function. However, for those who spend sufficient time barefoot, reduction in foot function is not seen to the extent it is in people who spend too much time in shoes.

Softer, cushioned shoes, such as those used for casual wear and many exercise shoes can cause balance problems in many people compared to shoes that are thinner and harder. Today's popular sports shoes are much thicker than even a few years ago. In those who jog or run, these types of shoes alter the gait for other reasons, too. Normally, both jogging and running are different than walking because of the way the foot hits the ground. When walking, we naturally move heel to toe—meaning we land on the back of our foot, the heel, and push off from the front of our foot. When jogging and running, we naturally land farther forward on our foot, more in the midfoot region; the faster pace causes us to land farther forward. We still push off similarly from the front of our foot. In popular sports shoes, we are forced to land on our heels during jogging and running, which is unnatural and a biomechanical hazard. Other activities, especially those requiring balance and delicate movement, require us to function in a similar fashion.

Joggers and runners who wear popular running shoes must contract their tibialis anterior muscle more than they normally would during each step in order to land on their heels. During natural running, with a very flat shoe or when barefoot, this constant high level of tibialis anterior muscle contraction does not have to take place. This excessive muscle contraction could result in overfacilitation of this muscle, with the potential for abnormal inhibition of the tibialis posterior muscle or other patterns of imbalance. In cases where the problem is chronic, the tibialis anterior muscle can fatigue itself and become inhibited. In addition, gastrocnemius and soleus muscle tightness can be a secondary problem, with tightness in the Achilles tendon. In any of these situations, the resulting muscle imbalance can lead to common injuries. The exact area of injury can vary from person to person since we all have different feet.

In addition, wearing today's shoes cause many to jog or run with an abnormally *longer* stride length, which further contributes to an abnormal gait. This, in turn, results in an abnormally high impact through the feet, with additional stress through the knees. Up to a third of injuries seen in runners and joggers are in the area of the knee, and this may be one common cause.

When discussing the potential of many types of shoes to cause harm, we can sum it up in two words: Consumer beware! Be especially aware of the hype associated with the product, and realize the most natural and safe position for the foot is without a shoe. The information in Chapter 8 will help you find shoes that will protect your feet from potential hazards on the road but allow your feet to be themselves.

8

BUYING THE RIGHT SHOES

The correct shoe should feel almost perfect on your foot. It should also wear well, keep its shape over time, tread safely, allow for sufficient foot freedom, minimally distort the foot, and hold together for a long time.

These characteristics depend on the quality of materials; the manufacturing process, including how the shoe was put together; and how well each shoe matches the structure of your foot. In general, the best shoes are those that are flattest, and those made specifically for your feet. Unfortunately, most people buy off-the-shelf shoes, so it's very important for follow strict guidelines for optimal fit.

In addition to proper shoe fit, certain shoe styles are inherently good or bad. For example, no matter how well a fancy, high-heeled shoe with a small toe box is made, it is still bad for your foot. Today, virtually all people know this. But many former high-heel wearers and millions of others are now buying sports shoes, which can also be harmful, as discussed in the previous chapter.

Considering that your feet are probably two different sizes, shoe-size numbers (for example size "10" or size "7") have no real meaning, and most companies don't have consistent sizes, so finding the optimal shoe may be more difficult than running a marathon. However, there are a number of things you can do to eliminate common dangers and find the best match for your feet. The most important factor is fit.

FINDING YOUR FIT

Optimal shoe fit may be difficult for some people, while others have an easy time. Research shows there are thirty-eight different factors associated with shoe fit. In addition to length and width, many other factors are subjective. This makes most shoes difficult to fit properly.

Poor shoe fit is the most common problem associated with shoe wear. If you take your health seriously, give your feet the time and attention they need. Skimp on style not fit.

The majority of people in the Western world probably wear shoes that are too small. Certainly in my practice, where, for more than twenty years I looked at every patient's shoes and feet, that was the case. In many situations, I would measure the foot and the shoe to show patients how poorly their shoe fit their foot. Other studies have shown the same common problem—that most people wear shoes that are too small. The reason women have more foot problems than men is due to the fact that more women don't fit into their shoes well.

A continual hindrance of optimal shoe fit is the absence of a standard shoe-size system. The ability to obtain accurate measurements of the foot has existed for more than three hundred years. As part of the job-protection measures many craftsmen took in early times, shoes were individually coded. Shoemakers marked the inside of the shoe with their personal codes that deliberately kept the size a secret from the customers and virtually ensured their return for new shoes. This is still in evidence today, as many manufacturers maintain individual size systems to promote customer loyalty.

Today's shoe sizes include three popular but different length-sizing systems, depending on where the shoes were made. These systems include sizing for shoes made in the United Kingdom, which originated in the late 1600s, the United States, which originated in the late 1800s, and continental or Paris Point metric, which originated in the late 1600s. Other sizing systems exist. More recently, the Mostro Point system was proposed to replace all other systems. This system is based on a simple length and width measurement in millimeters. It would be a great benefit to consumers, but it will probably never be accepted by the shoe industry since it would detract from the ability of shoe companies to sell more shoes.

MEASURING YOUR FEET

Most adults don't measure their feet when buying new shoes, especially considering that many shoe purchases today are online. As a result, many people squeeze into the same shoe size for years, or even decades. As previously discussed, adult feet stop growing by age twenty, but they still get larger through the years—sometimes by more than two sizes. They also get larger as the day goes on, returning to "normal" by the next morning, so always measure your feet and try on new shoes at the end of the day. Combine this with the fact that units of measure for shoes are not consistent, and you can easily get frustrated and not want to take the time needed to find the best fit.

Consider U.S. shoes. A shoe marked size 10 may be made differently from another shoe that's also marked size 10. Both actually will measure different lengths. Still another pair of size 10 shoes made with a different manufacturing method can measure differently than the other two size 10s. Actually, it's possible that a shoe marked size 10 could be one of five different sizes. So much for that silver gadget, called the *Brannock device* (see Figure 8.1), that shoe stores use to measure your feet. In addition, shoes for men, women, and children have different size units—a size 8 men's shoe is much different in length than a size 8 women's shoe.

The three popular size systems don't have much in common either. In the United States, a men's size 10 is the same in Canada, but in the United Kingdom it's a size 9. The same size in Japan is 27.5, and the continental equivalent is size 43.

In addition to length, width is a very important dimension. The width is measured across the ball of the foot. Add *height* to the foot and you have volume as another important measurement that is usually neglected. An example of the complexity of shoe fit is with volume, which is best assessed by foot comfort when trying out shoes on a hard floor.

By now you may be thinking that this is complicated. It is. But since there's no standard for size, none of these numbers should really mean anything to you, with one exception: fit.

MEASURING DEVICES

One benefit of measuring your feet is keep track of their *relative size.* This may not relate to shoe size. The Brannock device was introduced in 1927 with the purpose of providing a starting point for shoe fitting, not to dictate the best shoe size.

By using either the Brannock device in a shoe store, or doing the measuring yourself as described below, you could, and should, keep track of your foot size just like you would keep track of your weight with a scale or your overall health with a regular blood test. Like most health-related tests, measuring your feet is merely a general guide.

Any measurement of your feet should be done in a standing position on a hard floor. Do this at the end of the day, since most people's feet are slightly larger then, compared to the morning. Any meaningful daily size fluctuations must be differentiated from serious health problems, such as edema and certain pathological changes.

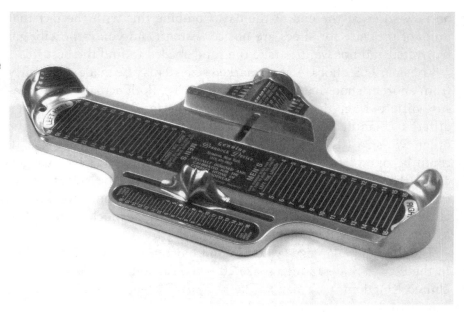

For an accurate measurement, make a footprint. Use a wet foot on a paper towel, or draw the outline of your foot with a pencil. Measure the back of the heel to the end of the big toe, in each foot. The purpose for this would be to see how much your feet change from year to year, not to relate it to any shoe size.

10 STEPS TO A BETTER FIT

Without taking shoe sizes very seriously, you can still get the best fit by following some key points:

1. Never assume you'll take the same size as your previous shoe, even if it's the same type or model. Rely on fit and comfort rather than any particular size.
2. Always plan on spending adequate time when shopping for shoes. Don't rush; if you're short on time, postpone it and set time aside for this important event. You may not find the right shoe in the first store you visit. Most outlets carry only a few of the many shoes in the marketplace.
3. Always try on both shoes. First, try on the size you think would fit best. Even if that size feels fine, try on a half-size larger. If that one feels the same, or even better, try on another half-size larger. Many people don't realize that a larger shoe may actually feel and fit better.
4. Continue trying on larger half-sizes until you find the shoes

that are obviously too large. Then go back to the previous half-size. More often than not that's the pair that best matches your feet. There should be at least a half-inch between your longest toe and the front of the shoe.

5. Each time you try on a pair of shoes, find a hard surface to walk on rather than the thick, soft carpet in shoe stores, where almost any shoe will feel good. If there's no sturdy floor to walk on, ask if you can walk outside (if you're not allowed, shop elsewhere).

6. You may also need to try different widths to get the best fit. The ball of your foot should fit comfortably into the widest part of the shoe, without causing the shoe to bulge.

7. Use comfort as the main criteria. Many salespeople are aware of how to find the right shoe size, and many are not. Don't let anyone tell you that you have to break in the shoes before they feel good. The best shoes for you are the ones that feel good right away. Often, shoes from mail-order outlets cost less, but be prepared to ship them back if they don't fit just right.

8. If the difference between your two feet is less than a half-size, fit the larger foot. If you have a significant difference of more than a half-size between your feet, it may be best to wear two different-sized shoes. How you accomplish this is up to you.

9. For sports shoes, many women fit better in men's shoes than in women's. The first rule, though, is that the shoe must fit properly. Some women don't fit into men's shoes, and some stores don't carry or companies don't make men's shoes in sizes that are small enough for many women.

10. Remember that the manufacturer makes new shoes based on trends of style, color, and fancy gimmicks to market the shoe. That's why shoe styles come and go. If you find the shoe that fits perfectly, buy more than one pair. Just be sure to try them all on, since the same shoe may also vary in size.

Some patients I have seen bought larger shoes after their initial problem of a tight fit was identified, only to find that their feet kept getting larger. At some point, they ended up with an increase of a whole size or more. I have even seen increases in adults of two and a half sizes over a two-year period!

SOCKS

When trying on shoes, wear the socks you would normally wear with them. Socks are not necessary but are mainly for added comfort. Like shoes, socks can be too tight, contributing to foot stress. For most situations, socks should be thin and not tight. Thick socks may require a half-size larger shoe.

GOOD SHOE, BAD SHOE

Not all shoes are harmful. But the vast majority of today's shoes can injure the feet. In general, the shoes that harm the foot the most are those that interfere with the foot's natural function. Virtually all shoes have the potential to do this. Of course, any shoe can injure the foot if it does not fit correctly.

The best shoes are those with little or no support, such as moccasins, sandals, flat sneakers, and shoes with thin and hard rather than soft soles. The worst shoes may be tight, high-heeled dress shoes and sports shoes with a thick sole that are also often filled with "special" materials, including air, and those that are extremely cushioned.

CATEGORIES OF SHOES

Below are the eight categories of shoes listed in Chapter 6 with very general comments about their potential to be good or bad for your feet.

- *Boots.* Because boots extend above the ankle, their potential to weaken the ankles over time is possible if the boot is too snug. The problem of ankle support is mentioned below with high-top sneakers, and discussed in Chapter 9. Heels that are more than about an inch above the rest of the foot can, over time, cause foot problems, leading to poor balance.
- *Clogs.* With thick soles, these shoes can also lead to poor balance.
- *Lace-ups.* These are the best regular casual, dress, and formal shoes for most people. However, the soles should not be too thick or heels too high (less than about one inch). Sports shoes used for casual wear and exercise have great potential for harm, as previously discussed. However, some models are available that are much more flat and do not have very thick heels (these are called *racing flats*). Nike, Adidas, New Balance, and many other companies make these. In addition, there are a variety of inexpensive flat sports shoes and sneakers that, with the proper fit, can be very good shoes for casual use and exercise. These are discussed below.
- *Moccasins.* Whether very light and flimsy, or as thin-soled loafers, moccasins can be very good casual and dress shoes for most people.

- *Monks.* Like the lace-up shoes, these may be good if the soles are thin and heels not more than about one inch thick.
- *Mules.* These may be good shoes when the heels are an inch or less.
- *Pumps.* These high-heeled shoes are potentially the most dangerous, along with sports shoes. If your feet are healthy, you could get away with an occasional brief evening of wear without too much risk.
- *Sandals.* Flat sandals can be good shoes for most people.

For more information about children's shoes, see Chapter 16. Sports shoes are further addressed here because these shoes are so prominent today and have such potential impact on the feet.

SPORTS SHOES

They used to be called just sneakers, but today's version is the athletic, running, or sports shoe. More of these shoes are worn by nonathletes, and even more by those who don't exercise at all. Almost everyone in the Western world has at least one pair, from infants just learning to walk to the elderly who have unsteady gaits. Many athletes have several pairs. Consumers buy these shoes by the hundreds of millions.

These shoes tend to be much thicker than they were a few years ago, and thicker than most other shoes due to the added materials. These may include a thicker sole, air pockets, a thicker midsole, and a thicker insert.

The reason these shoes are so popular is marketing. Billions of dollars have been spent to convince the consumer that today's sports shoes can perform seemingly miraculous feats. These include improving balance, running faster, reducing injuries, absorbing shock, and otherwise improving foot function. The fact is most advertising claims are not true.

Then there's the issue of style. It's cool to wear the latest trend, or have the same shoes a famous sports figure wears. Actually, the sports figure probably does not wear anything like an off-the-shelf sports shoe. If these shoes are not good enough for a professional athlete, why should you wear them?

Many people believe that expensive running shoes are the perfect casual shoe. After all, if they protect you during running, they must be perfect for just standing around and lounging. This, of course, is not necessarily true. Then there's the issue of our teens vying for the best shoes on the block. And, casual joggers and runners want what they think are the best, no matter what the price. If the only problem with these shoes *was* price, I would not be writing about it.

Joggers and runners wear many sports shoes. Of the millions of people who jog or run worldwide, more than half are injured within any given year. In comparison, barefoot runners, and there are many of them worldwide, are rarely injured.

The best shoes for jogging and running are those that are flat, with a heel close to the level of the rest of the foot. Today, these are found in the category of racing flats. They're not just for racers but anyone who wants a shoe that does not have as much potential to do harm. Much less expensive versions of these shoes can be found in some department stores and other popular outlets. Look for less fancy shoes without the gimmicks and you'll get a shoe that's fully functional with less potential for injury. Some can be found for $20 and even less than $10.

The same basic principles apply to other sports shoes. These include cleats, spikes, and other special shoes used in soccer, football, baseball, track and field, and golf.

"HIGH-TOP" SHOES

The most popular "high top" sports shoe in this category is the basketball sneaker. Plain high-top sneakers were popular for many years, but today they have become fancy, oversupported, overpriced high-top shoes.

Supposedly, the added ankle support, the key feature of this shoe, protects against ankle sprain and other injuries. But studies don't verify this. Actually, these shoes may do just the opposite, as basketball players may have the highest rates of ankle sprains of any sport. In addition, high-tops *increase* shock transmission, *reduce* jumping ability (reduce the height jumped), and *slow* running times relative to low-support shoes.

When the ankle, or any area of the body, is supported, we run the risk of weakening the area. This is the result of muscles that no longer have to work as much, losing some of their strength. Support around a joint, such as the ankle, does not really physically support the joint. This issue is further discussed in Chapter 9.

CUSTOM SHOES

Perhaps the best shoes are those made specifically to fit your foot. You can dictate the exact fit for each foot, the appropriate shoe volume, the sole you want, and a higher quality material such as leather. Unfortunately, this craft became nearly extinct, but today it's possible to find shoemakers who can produce a custom shoe to match your foot. An Internet search for custom shoes brings many sources. A local shoemaker would probably be best for getting precise measurements and service.

WEANING OFF BAD SHOES

If you've been reading this book and realize it's time to make a healthy change for your feet, you may have to go through a "withdrawal" from bad shoes to good shoes. It might be impossible to stop wearing bad shoes one day and start with good ones the next. The reason has to do with the position of your feet, specifically your muscles. Let's take the case of wearing high-heeled dress shoes. If you've been wearing these shoes five days a week for years, your foot muscles and tendons have changed in length. In addition, the ligaments have adapted, too. When suddenly you start wearing a flatter shoe, your muscles, tendons, and ligaments will have to re-adapt. This process may be uncomfortable, sometimes painful, if you try to do it all at once.

In making the change, you may feel discomfort right away or it could take a day or two. If your feet have more significant unnatural changes in the bones and joints, such as hammertoes or a bunion, the problem could be worse and take longer. For many people, these changes need to take place slowly if they are going to make the transition without much discomfort.

Even those who wear the popular thick-soled sports shoes may have become "addicted" to the supporting features of these shoes. In many cases, the muscles have become weak and will require a period of strengthening, which could happen during normal movement in good shoes. This is further discussed in Chapter 11.

For these and other shoe problems, making the change to flat shoes or even being barefoot, as natural as that is, makes your foot feel rather odd and often painful. This does not mean that being barefoot is a stressful state, but rather your feet have changed because of the kinds of shoes you've worn.

For many people, weaning off bad shoes may take at least one extra step. First, look at the highest heel height of a current shoe. Compare this to a lower heel or a flat shoe. Your first step in weaning off bad shoes is to wear a shoe that's about half to three-quarters less in height than the height of the one you currently wear. Try wearing a shoe with this height of heel for a few days to make sure your feet don't become painful. If there is pain, you'll require two extra steps and have to wean slower by wearing shoes whose heels are only one-quarter to half the height of what you're used to wearing before going to one that is half to three-quarters.

Whether you need to take one or two steps in making the transition from bad to good shoes, it may only take a month or two to make the appropriate adaptations to the new foot position. For others, it could take as long as six months. Rely on the feet feeling good for at least a week or two before progressing to the next step. Once you've weaned down to more flat shoes, you'll wonder how you survived the others.

OLD SHOES

It's been said that old worn shoes can be bad. This may be true if your old shoes were bad to start with. A good shoe that has a lot of wear may still be good. Properly made shoes that match your feet should last many years. Even sports shoes can last a long time before they need to be retired. Marketing has made many people believe that we have to replace our shoes frequently. This may be true when the shoes are poorly made, but even cheap shoes can last a long time.

A number of factors may cause you to either repair or replace your current shoes. First and foremost, they should remain comfortable. As soon as they cease being comfortable, they need to be repaired or replaced.

Another factor is wear. The two heaviest areas of wear are the heel and under the ball of the foot. If your shoes wear very unevenly, this could be a problem. For example, if one heel is worn a quarter inch more than the other, this can cause a significant mechanical imbalance. The *cause* of this excess wear may be mechanical imbalance to start with. If one heel is worn down much more than the other, repair both heels if possible, or buy new shoes. If the area under the ball of the foot is worn through the sole, this is also a reason to repair or replace the shoe. In this case, a new sole may be needed.

A common problem in some shoes is the breakdown of the stiffener in the heel area. This is especially troublesome when the heel height is more than about an inch thick. This can create instability in the feet and lead to balance problems.

Some shoes get too stretched out after long periods of wear. This is especially true of loafers or shoes that don't lace up. If this is the case, your feet may be working hard to keep the shoes from coming off during movement. This is accomplished with constant increased muscle contraction, which can lead to muscle imbalance.

Most of these problems result in some level of discomfort. However, many people get used to a shoe being uncomfortable, so sometimes the discomfort is not obvious.

COSTS

We could not have a complete discussion about *buying* shoes without addressing costs. Most popular shoes cost between $40 and $100. For growing teens, fashion-oriented consumers, athletes, and many others who buy shoes frequently or wear them out relatively quickly, or anyone who sees shoe prices as absurd or unfair, an alternative is appreciated.

First, cost and fit have nothing in common, with the only possible exception being custom shoes. Likewise, cost may have nothing in common with quality or support, either. In fact, one study demonstrated that in comparison to the cheapest shoes, the more expensive sports shoes are actually associated with more than twice the injury rate.

There are many low-cost, high-quality shoes on the market that sell for much less than the hyped brands. For women, a pair of flat Keds is great for casual wear, but they're no longer made for men. A shoe called Silver Series from Wal-Mart works well for men and costs less than $10. Flat sandals and moccasins, including loafers, can also be very inexpensive, look good, and last a long time.

A good choice if you want to spend more money on a stylish shoe is the Puma Mostro and similar models. They're flat, not supported, and your friends will love them.

If you're into gimmicks, styles, or just have to have the latest trend, you'll pay a lot for shoes that may not last very long. Shoe companies count on that. For dress or formal occasions, the right fitting shoe will last a long time—almost a lifetime if you have them stretched when you need more room. A well-made shoe can be stretched as needed, although there are limits.

Cost factors are especially a concern when buying shoes for kids, whose feet are always growing. On one end of the spectrum, you don't want to interfere with the child's growing foot, since this is the time when many foot problems can start. On the other end, companies market heavily to youngsters who ask (or demand) the latest trends. Unfortunately, once kids see enough shoe commercials on TV, they'll want only the expensive ones. Train them early or suffer the consequences. Or, get them the basics but let them buy the extras. Children's feet and their shoes are discussed in Chapter 16.

My Shoes

Whether it's diet, nutrition, exercise, or other lifestyle factors, many of my patients and others who know me often ask about my habits. In the case of shoes, it's easy to answer. I spend the majority of my time barefoot. This includes exercise most of the time. If my exercise brings me to places other than the hard flat sand of the beach, I wear flat, low-cut All Stars (sneakers for about $25) or Silver Series, and I recently started using Puma Mostros. When I go into town, I wear very flat sandals or moccasins, leather made, and have flat lace-ups for dress occasions or formal wear. I have very good-looking footwear, and my average new purchase is about once every three years.

When buying shoes also consider what's in them (such as supports) and lacing. You'll learn more about these in the next chapter.

9

FOOT SUPPORT AND LACING

Many shoes have built-in or removable supports, but in addition to these, many companies have developed a wide array of shoe devices. The first big business for these products, New Balance Arch and Support Company, was founded in Boston in 1906.

These supports are made for the heel, sole, arch, and ankle and include soft and hard materials comprised of cotton, leather, synthetics, plastic, wood, and metal. They come in the form of heel and sole supports, ankle braces, a variety of inserts and arch supports including orthotics, and others.

In addition to conventional supports, many forms of taping are used, especially in sports, to help support the foot and ankle. In my twenty-year experience using conservative treatments for many types of foot problems, successful outcome does not require any type of support in the vast majority of cases. Only on occasion would additional foot support be necessary and almost always for a very short period, during which time the foot can heal.

In rare situations, long-term support may be necessary. Also, stabilizing or immobilizing the foot or ankle may be necessary in an emergency, when the risk of serious damage is suspected, and until such time as a proper assessment can be made. Such situations, which are very individual in nature, are not detailed in this book.

However, the long-term use of foot supports by the average consumer is very common for treating mild or moderate complaints, or when added support is not necessary. Despite the potential risk, these items are heavily marketed and readily available in many retail outlets and online sites. In addition, even though these items come in different sizes and shapes, they are essentially "one size fits all," since they usually don't specifically match the needs of the individual foot, despite what the manufacturer says.

Some people use these devices for a very short period without success, only to try one type after another, with many supports ending up in the drawer unused. If you don't specifically match a particular support to your precise needs, it could lead to long-term worsening of the condition, making proper treatment much more difficult.

The use of foot supports is very common. However, there are risks associated with supporting the foot when such treatment is not truly required. In most cases, the use of shoe supports should be considered only after more conservative therapy has been tried and is without success, and before more radical treatment, such as surgery, is considered.

HOW SUPPORTS CAN WEAKEN THE FOOT

The greatest harm from the use of foot supports is that through their routine use the need for other more appropriate treatments that address the cause of the problem may be overlooked. This is especially true when supports provide temporary symptomatic relief, giving the false impression that the problem is solved.

In some cases, a support will provide symptomatic relief in the area that is painful, only to trigger discomfort in another area previously not a problem. For example, you may start using a particular support that provides relief from your foot pain. A week later, your knee may begin to hurt. This can occur as a result of the initial change made in the structure of your foot by the support, thus causing other structural changes—sometimes up the leg into the knee, hip, or even low back.

Supporting a joint when it is not required can actually increase the risk of injury to that joint. This is true not only for the foot and ankle, but for any joint such as the knee, hip, or those of the low back. The reason is that the added support can reduce muscle function leading to muscle imbalance. With the additional support, our foot's natural internal support gives way to the external support with the result of reduced muscle function. In other words, our foot muscles have no reason to work as much since something else (the added support) is doing the job for them. And no support can ever take the place of proper muscle function.

In many cases, a foot support can reduce the ranges of motion in the joints. Reduced ranges of motion can lead to joint and muscle dysfunction and increase the risk for injuries due to minor twists or turns that normally would not be problematic. In certain instances, reduced ranges of motion may be necessary to assist in healing, such as after an ankle sprain. However, it's important to remove the support as the body completes the healing process to prevent a continuation of lowered ranges of motion and allow for the foot to strengthen its muscles and return to normal.

Even when a support is necessary, a softer or semirigid support such as leather, rather than a hard or rigid support such as plastic, usually works best and may even quicken the healing process. This may also apply to the case of a foot fracture, where a semirigid rather than a rigid support is usually best. However, these more serious conditions must be treated individually.

ARCH SUPPORTS

The notion that our arches need support is incorrect. They work just fine in their own natural state as evident from our evolution, during which humans have been mostly barefoot. Today, our foot naturally still has a higher arch when not bearing weight, and it flattens out considerably with weight bearing. This is especially true in those who spend a lot of time barefoot and have maintained healthy arch function. Some people confuse this normal flattening with "flat feet" or a pronation problem.

As discussed earlier, the arches of the foot are supported and maintained by muscles. The medial arch is very important, with the tibialis posterior being the key muscle. Disturbance of muscle function due to shoe problems can lead to an abnormal inhibition of this muscle, resulting in medial arch dysfunction. In this common situation, addressing the cause of the muscle problem should be the primary treatment rather than using an arch support to take the place of the muscle's normal activity.

A common cause of tibialis posterior and other muscle dysfunction is wearing improper shoes, especially those that are too thick and oversupported. The reduced foot-sense also interferes with normal muscle function.

Many shoes come with supports that can be removed. Some can be easily taken out while other may require a little pulling. These are very general supports that usually don't match the specific needs of your foot. In most cases, you're better off removing as much as possible from the shoe. In addition to allowing your foot to function more freely, the shoe will become thinner and more firm, both healthy attributes.

ORTHOTICS

The use of an orthotic device should not be a first line of therapy for most foot problems. This is not to discount the potential benefits of these devices for a very small number of people. One potential problem with the use of orthotics is that the need for other therapies may be overlooked. People who have past or current surgical needs, who have suffered a stroke, or who for various reasons will never have normal foot function are more difficult or even impossible to treat using only a conservative approach. In these cases, orthotics can be useful.

Orthotics and other similar inserts, including those with shock-absorbing abilities, have not been shown to protect against the risks of injury. These devices may actually further reduce arch function and provide excessive cushioning, which can increase the risk of injury. Orthotics are often prescribed to patients with knee pain. However, studies have not shown this to be effective. In addition, electromyographic studies fail to show any significant differences in the average muscle activity of the tibialis anterior, peroneus longus, and gastrocnemius muscles when orthotics are used.

Placing orthotics in your shoes most often results in the shoe fitting differently, usually too tightly. In this instance, the shoe must either be modified or a different shoe used. Unfortunately, this is not normally done and many people with added support have ill-fitting shoes.

Many orthotics are made to order—at least that's what the consumer is told. However, most orthotics are not custom made to *your* foot but to a general model of an average foot. Those who have their foot measured or cast to find the best fit should understand that a cast of the dysfunctional foot is being used to make the orthotics, and these devices may just maintain your foot in the original unbalanced position. Balancing the foot first, then measuring or casting it is the ideal approach.

Many orthotics are made from hard materials such as plastic and sometimes even metal. I could never understand these materials for use in a person without a serious permanent condition, as these materials are often used on many functional problems. Your foot moves through many ranges of motion during the course of standing, walking, or running. The best material to use is leather because it will move with the foot.

HEEL LIFTS

The use of heel lifts has been popular for many years. These are often recommended for plantar fasciitis, Achilles tendon pain, or the so-called short-leg syndrome said to contribute to low back and other pains. Because they may provide some symptomatic relief does not mean the cause of the problem has been found. Like other supports, even if you feel better with lifts, the cause of the problem is usually not addressed.

Heel lifts can make structural changes in the feet, ankle, legs, pelvis, and spine. However, studies show that the use of heel lifts can also result in increased impact and increased instability of the foot. The result can be a higher weight-bearing stress on the joints in the foot and ankle and possibly on the knees, hips, and pelvis, too.

Heel lifts may provide relief of symptoms in a variety of problems:

- Heel lifts may temporarily improve symptoms of plantar pain. However, in the process, other areas of the foot and ankle may become mechanically stressed.

- Some people use heel lifts to attempt to improve low back pain. It's clear that heel lifts can change the posture of the pelvis and low back. However, whether this change makes a real improvement of the problem, no change or a worsening of the problem is left to chance.

- For those with a so-called short-leg syndrome, heel lifts are sometimes recommended. However, if the "short leg" is functional, which is almost always the case, and any discomfort or pain is due to muscle imbalance and not to a true shortening of the leg, heel lifts are not the best remedy since they do not address the problem. For those with a history of a broken bone in the leg or thigh resulting in a true or *anatomical* short leg (other causes exist, too), a heel lift may be helpful since one leg is truly shorter than the other.

- Heel lifts are sometimes used for those with Achilles tendon pain. This is due to the elevated heel reducing the activity of the gastrocnemius muscle, thereby reducing tension in the Achilles tendon. However, in some cases, gastrocnemius muscle function is already diminished and is one of the causes of the problem.

- The temporary use of heel lifts may be important after certain surgical conditions, such as in postoperative management of a ruptured Achilles tendon.

TAPING

Mild taping of the ankle and foot may help prevent injuries, but not through immobilization. Mild taping involves two or three strips of tape attaching to the lower leg, ankle, and around the foot. This may prevent injuries by stimulating the nerve endings in the skin, thus helping the muscles perform better. The tape tractions or pulls on the skin, providing increased foot-sense to better allow the nervous system to adapt to movement. This simple technique is described in Chapter 11.

Mildly taping the foot and ankle may help prevent injury by significantly restoring impaired foot-sense caused by shoe wear. This actually may be the primary benefit of taping, since any real support function is lost after as few as twenty minutes.

Heavier taping, common in sports, can reduce foot range of motion and impair athletic performance. These effects include reduced speed, agility, and jumping ability.

ELASTIC SUPPORT

The popular use of elastic support is different from taping. These supports don't have much effect on foot-sense presumably because they don't "stick" to the skin like tape and have much less of an effect on the nerves within. Studies have shown that compared to other devices, elastic supports were much less effective in treating various foot and ankle conditions. Like other supports, elastic devices can cause muscle dysfunction if worn for too long.

LACING

Some shoe problems are not due to fit but poor lacing technique. How difficult can it be to tie your shoes? After all, we learned how to do that a long time ago. Well, the fact is that many people don't lace their shoes correctly, and sometimes it can make a significant difference in how a shoe fits. In addition, many people don't tie their laces, making the shoe fit too loose–an unstable situation for anyone.

Sometimes lacing too tightly is sufficient enough stress to cause problems. Lacing should be snug–not too loose but not tight. There should never be discomfort associated with lacing or any discomfort under the area of the laces. The most important aspect of lacing is that after tying your shoes, they should be completely comfortable, and after they've been on for a while, they should be just as comfortable. This should be true for not only the laces but also the whole shoe.

There are many different types of lacing used for many different types of shoes by different types of shoe wearers. Using comfort as your guide, you'll always get the best fit. Here are some general tips to lace more effectively:

- Always lace from the toes upward, beginning with the holes or *eyelets* farthest down.
- For each set of eyelets you go through with the lace, pull the lace snug so the same amount of tension is evenly distributed through the lace.
- Use a crisscross or zigzag pattern–most people and most shoes function best with this approach (see Figure 9.1a and b, below).

■ When you finish lacing, all areas of the lace should have the same tension.

The crisscross style of lacing is the most common way to tie shoes in the United States. In Europe, it's more common to use straight lacing, where instead of all the laces going up the shoe in a diagonal pattern, some go from hole to hole straight across. It's been shown that both the crisscross and European patterns are equally effective. If either of these patterns of lacing is not comfortable, it's most likely that the shoe itself does not fit correctly.

In addition, the crisscross pattern requires the least amount of lace, so you'll always have sufficient lace for tying. The European style is the second-most efficient approach for lace use.

If you have a very irregular foot, you may require any number of different types of lacing, so choose one that matches your particular needs. In this case, you may also be wearing special shoes, and a specialist should be able to help with lacing. In any situation, don't be afraid to experiment but always use the comfort factor as the ultimate index.

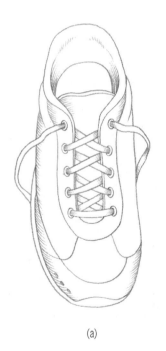

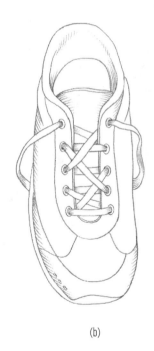

(a)   (b)

FIGURE 9.1 The two most common lacing styles: American (a), and European (b).

With a better understanding of basic foot anatomy and movement—and the ability to assess your problems—you are ready to move on to treatment topics in the next section.

SECTION THREE

TREATMENT

After assessing your foot problem, you may decide to use certain conservative remedies to correct the problem. These range from rest and ice to hands-on therapies such as acupressure, massage, and similar treatments, and biochemical remedies such as diet and nutrition. In addition, for those with significant discomfort, simple pain control techniques can be very effective.

The traditional approach to treating most problems is to first name the condition. You've already noticed this is not the approach I've taken. Rather, improving function should be your therapeutic goal. If you improve the function of the foot–get everything inside working properly– almost any problem will be corrected.

This section discusses a variety of natural remedies the average person can use for improving foot function. Perhaps the most successful, easiest, and most natural remedy for many foot problems is going barefoot.

1 0

BEING BAREFOOT

If you really want to be free, be barefoot. Not only are your feet made for walking, they're made to do it barefoot. As a bonus, for those with foot problems, it's also the best and quickest way to rehabilitate your feet.

Without the restriction of shoes, your foot muscles can ultimately return to their natural state of optimal function. In some people, this could take time. For example, if you're used to wearing high-heeled shoes or thick-soled sports shoes most of the time, being barefoot will be a big transition. But once you experience the freedom of being bare, you'll wonder how you got by without it.

Baring the soles may be difficult for some, not just physically but mentally and emotionally, too. After all, we're taught by society that being barefoot is somehow dirty or low class. Yes, when you walk barefoot your soles will get dirty. But you'll track less dirt compared to wearing shoes—you'll actually look where you're walking when barefoot and avoid stepping on things you don't think about when wearing shoes—and your feet won't have any more germs than your hands or mouth.

For those who need support—not the type in the shoes but mental and emotional support—consider the Dirty Sole Society (www.barefooters. org), Barefoot Runners (www.barefootrunners.org), Parents for Barefoot Children (www.unshod.org/pfbc), and the many other groups that promote healthy barefoot living. We are not alone.

Physically, making the transition to bare feet will involve toughening up your soles. This sometimes makes people uneasy, but consider that the more time spent barefoot, the fewer calluses you'll have. Even though your soles may get tougher, you won't notice it except in being able to walk or even exercise barefoot almost anywhere without discomfort. Even though you'll have tougher soles, you'll actually have *more* sensation in your feet as a result of being barefoot.

The state of being barefoot is referred to as *unshod* (referring to unshoed), while wearing shoes is called *shod.*

BAREFOOT THERAPY

If you still need an excuse to go barefoot, do it for your health. You can even tell people you're undergoing special rehabilitation by order of the doctor. The fact is, being barefoot can help restore normal muscle function in the feet better than any other therapy. It accomplishes this by allowing normal movement and improving foot-sense.

As discussed earlier, making the transition from high-heeled or thick, oversupported shoes can be difficult. In some cases, you may have to "wean" off the worst of shoes. But for many people, being barefoot, or unshod, is not a physical stress. If that is true for you, you can start right now.

If you're not used to being barefoot, start by walking unshod around your home. It's best without socks, but a thin pair would be acceptable if your feet get cold. Walk on the bare floor, carpeted areas, basement cement, and any other surfaces available. Different surfaces will provide different types of stimulation for your bare feet, and that's what you're looking for—a variety of stimulation to restore normal foot-sense.

If you have not ventured outdoors after a couple of weeks, take the plunge. This will provide much more foot stimulation because the ground is uneven and not smooth like your indoor surfaces. Walking on grass, dirt, sand, and other natural surfaces will provide great motivation for your feet to improve foot-sense. Even your driveway, sidewalk, and porch can provide additional types of stimulus for your feet.

I've spent many of my days outdoors barefoot and have never sustained cuts or injury other than the occasional minor scrapes. Conversely, I have had several occurrences of serious injury while wearing shoes during outdoor activities.

After a few more weeks of being barefoot, especially with outdoor activity, your foot function should be improving and your feet should feel better. During this period, you should also be wearing shoes that fit properly and better match your feet. This may mean buying new ones and also disposing of the ones that don't fit. Unlike clothing, don't keep your tight-fitting shoes thinking your feet will someday get smaller. They won't.

Where you go from here with your newfound freedom is up to you. Despite what most people think, and what the signs in some restaurant and shop windows say, it's not illegal to enter public places barefoot. Some retailers may not want you in their store barefoot, but that's *their* rule. Despite what they may say, it's not against any health department regulations. Nor is it illegal to drive barefoot.

Once you've established better foot function through healthy barefoot adaptation, it's important to maintain two habits: First, spend as much time as possible being barefoot throughout the year. Even when the weather is bad, being barefoot indoors virtually all the time can help maintain proper foot function. Second, once you've weaned off bad shoes and restored good foot function, be careful not to return to old bad habits by wearing bad shoes, with the only exception perhaps being the occasional dressy event.

There are many exercise programs and equipment available to improve foot function, but most won't accomplish any more than the benefits obtained by being barefoot. If your foot problems require more help than barefoot rehabilitation, the next chapter discusses some traditional remedies.

11

TRADITIONAL REMEDIES

In addition to being barefoot, a number of other remedies may be useful for the rehabilitation of many foot and ankle problems. These include the use of hot and cold, the two most popular and longtime home remedies. Also, rolling the plantar muscles with a golf ball, strengthening specific muscles that have weakened, and a simple method of taping to improve foot-sense are discussed.

While many of these remedies can be very effective, nothing is as effective overall as being barefoot, with the exception of cold applications for acute injuries. Therefore, to obtain the best results, the utilization of remedies discussed in this chapter should be performed *in addition* to barefoot therapy, except in situations where rest is necessary.

These remedies are for home use. In some cases, professional help may be necessary and may include other more specific remedies that address your particular problem.

ACUTE PROBLEMS

For acute foot problems–those injuries that have occurred recently, such as a fall, twisted ankle, or stubbed toe–the word to think of is *RICE*: *r*est, *i*ce, *c*ompression, and *e*levation.

- The benefits of *rest* have already been discussed. When your foot needs rest, nothing is better. Rest can prevent further damage following injury and give your body the time and energy it needs to heal.
- The use of *ice* is discussed below.

■ Mild *compression* can help reduce swelling, especially when there are broken blood vessels. Compression should be applied carefully, so as not to further traumatize the area. Even the weight of an ice pack can be enough compression.

■ *Elevation* refers to putting your foot up on your desk, lying on the floor with your foot on the couch, or lying in bed with your foot elevated with pillows. This helps prevent excess fluid from building up in the area of injury. If there are broken blood vessels, elevating the foot helps speed the repair process.

CRYOTHERAPY

The therapeutic use of cold is called *cryotherapy* or *hypothermia*. It is a form of counter-irritation, where the skin and areas just below it are irritated with very cold temperatures to stimulate healing. Like many therapies, ice can be very helpful when properly applied, but it can do harm if used incorrectly. Cooling an area of injury can help reduce inflammation and muscle tightness or spasm, both of which help reduce pain. In doing so, it can help speed the recovery process.

Ice is the most popular way to cool the foot, but ice should never be applied directly to the skin. Instead, use a *moist* cloth or towel on the skin with the ice applied on top of it. A moist towel helps transfer the cooling benefits whereas a dry one can partly insulate your skin from the cold. In this way, the cooling effect can reach all areas, including, possibly, the bones.

The ice can be placed in a plastic bag, with smaller pieces of ice working better than large ice cubes, or you can use a freezer gel pack. Be sure the gel pack is not leaking, which can be irritating to the skin. In an emergency, a package of frozen peas or other items in your freezer may work just fine.

Applying ice to your foot produces four stages of sensation you can easily differentiate. First, the area will become cool, and you will feel this cold effect immediately. Second, you will feel a prickling or itchy sensation, sometimes described as a burning itch. Following this you will get an achy feeling; in some cases this can become painful. The last stage is numbness—the point when you know it's time to immediately remove the ice.

Apply ice until you feel numbness, or for no more than about twenty minutes. When in doubt, remove the ice. The therapeutic effects occur in the early and mid-stages, and risk of ice injury increases in the later stage. You can apply the ice again once the skin temperature has returned to normal, although once every hour or two is sufficient for most situations.

In addition to using cold on the foot, cooling tight muscles in the leg can sometimes help the foot. For example, in cases of heel pain or Achilles tendon pain caused by tight gastrocnemius and soleus muscles, the use of cryotherapy on these leg muscles may be helpful. The other muscle group that commonly becomes tight is the plantar muscles on the bottom of the foot, where ice can also be used.

CONTRAINDICATIONS FOR ICE

Since the foot is not well endowed with large muscles or fat, the use of ice has the potential to cause harm. The overenthusiastic use of ice can literally freeze the skin and small blood vessels and injure nerves. Essentially, frostbite can result from the use of cryotherapy, unless it is applied with caution.

In many situations, ice is *not* indicated and should be avoided as it can further injure the foot. Those with rheumatoid arthritis, Raynaud's syndrome, or any type of paralysis should not use ice. Also avoid ice on areas of reduced sensation. Limit or avoid the use of ice over areas where a large nerve passes close to the skin surface, such as under the ankle bones on the inside and outside of the foot.

A very small number of people have *cold allergies* and can have adverse reactions to cold. Most people already know the condition exists because of previous adverse reactions to cold, including pain and skin rash. Those with high blood pressure should also be cautious when using ice as it can raise blood pressure.

Take care when using ice boots or other strap-on ice packs. Because they are so convenient to use, people often not only use them for too long a time but tend to be active during cryotherapy–itself a contraindication as rest and elevation are what is required. For obvious reasons, do not put these devices on before going to sleep.

For acute injuries, especially during the first twenty-four hours, certain remedies should be avoided. These include the use of heat in any form, whether a hot bath, heating pad, or heating gel. Heat can aggravate inflammation. An aggressive massage can also create heat and should be avoided. Stretching should not be used for acute problems.

Differentiating between the need for heat or cold is relatively easy–if your foot is hot, cool it; if cold, heat it. In general, cooling is the best therapy for acute problems. Cold therapy is easy to use and inexpensive but is often overlooked because of its simplicity.

COLD COMPRESSES

The benefits of cold need not always come from ice. An alternative is to use a towel soaked in very cold water with the excess water wrung out.

Keep the towel in the refrigerator to keep it very cold. This can have an excellent therapeutic effect as well, especially if a five-to-ten-minute application is all you require. Don't underestimate the benefits of this approach. It's also safer than the use of ice, which can have side effects.

COOL BATH

Another method of cooling the foot is a cold bath. This safer and effective form of cyrotherapy can be more therapeutic than using ice. A large bucket or small foot tub works well. Place your foot in cold water so it is completely submerged. Add enough ice to prevent the water from getting warm; do not fill the tub with ice. Depending on the temperature of the water, you can keep your foot immersed for five to twenty minutes. A deeper bath can also cool the muscles of the leg, which often influence the foot. A deep cold bath that cools the leg muscles is often the best way to improve overall function in the foot, and it can be more therapeutic than ice placed only on the area of discomfort.

While generally used for acute problems, a cold bath can be very helpful for chronic problems not associated with inflammation. A cold bath can improve muscle balance, especially if you can cover the leg up to the knee with cold water.

A moderately cold bath can also help recovery from exercise excess or even a day of wearing bad shoes. In this situation, your feet are tired and hot; even a five-minute cool bath can make your feet feel fresh and alive.

BLISTERS

A blister is a vesicle created by the separation of different layers of skin that fills with clear fluid, or sometimes blood. A blood blister forms when blood vessels within the blister are broken. It is due to a pinch bruise or constant friction, as is the case with poorly fitting shoes or walking barefoot too much before the skin has sufficiently adapted to the barefoot state. Most blisters occur on the bottoms of the feet and back heel area.

Moist skin produces blisters most easily, with very dry and very wet skin most protective against blister formation. Antiperspirants and powders don't prevent blisters, but acrylic socks may offer protection. Rather than look for products and materials that reduce blister incidence, it's best to obtain the best fitting shoes and socks, which are the best prevention against blisters.

There are two important factors regarding blisters. First, if you get one it means something is not right, and you need to find the cause of the problem. If the problem is improperly fitting shoes, change them immediately. Second, if you get a nontraumatic blister–such as the common types seen from poor shoe fit–it often precedes an injury. The blister is a sign that you have a significant imbalance. Making the necessary changes immediately can prevent further problems.

If you're new to barefoot walking and you get a blister, it may just be that your feet have not yet adapted by thickening the skin. In this case, wean yourself slower into barefoot walking.

Lightly puncturing the blister and draining it after a day may result in the best outcome and least discomfort, but be sure the area remains clean and free of chemicals.

CHRONIC PROBLEMS

A long-term foot problem may be more difficult to treat because the body has been unable to correct it. In some cases, a cold footbath, especially one that includes the whole leg up to the knee, can be very helpful. In other cases, heat may help correct a problem. For some people, certain muscles are too weak and need strengthening. For those who have worn bad shoes for a long period of time, specific *soft taping* of the foot can help rehabilitate it. Directing therapy at tight muscles may also help, such as in the case of tight plantar muscles.

HEAT

The use of heat therapy, sometimes called *thermotherapy* or *hyperthermia*, is one of the oldest home remedies. Warm and hot application can be comforting and emotionally relaxing. Various forms of heating are used from moist hot packs and hot baths to heating pads and hot gels. Moist heat is best as it penetrates better, whereas dry heat can dehydrate the skin.

Heat is generally reserved for more chronic conditions and usually is contraindicated in acute problems. Heat dilates the blood vessels within the foot. This allows improved circulation helping to bring in needed nutrients, including oxygen, and remove unwanted waste products.

Heat can also help reduce muscle tightness by relaxing or lengthening them. Unfortunately, unlike cold, heat can worsen muscles that are abnormally inhibited, since they are already lengthened too much. This is most often the case when heat is applied directly over the muscle.

One benefit of heat applications is pain reduction. This is especially true with heating gels or creams. This effect is not really therapeutic, but rather the heat stimulation on the skin fools the nervous system and pain is not felt as much by the brain. While this reduces pain, it can also eliminate your awareness of a problem and result in the potential for overuse.

CONTRAINDICATIONS OF HEAT

When in doubt about using heat, avoid it. You can too easily do more harm than good. Do not use heat when you have an acute injury. Avoid heat on an area that is inflamed, swollen, or bruised. In almost all these situations, the foot will feel warm–an indication to use cold, not hot. Also avoid heat with any skin disorder, diabetes, circulatory problem, or open wound. As mentioned above, heat can worsen an already abnormally inhibited muscle.

STRENGTHENING FOOT MUSCLES

Muscle weakness in the foot is common due to the types of shoes many people wear. The three-part exercise described below involves strengthening a variety of muscles that attach within the foot. These include the plantar muscles and the anterior and posterior tibialis muscles. Even if you have a problem in only one foot, it's best to exercise both feet. These are done best while sitting in a chair.

1. Place a dry cloth, towel, or sock flat on the floor. Place your bare foot on top of the sock. By contracting your plantar muscles, attempt to pick up the sock by squeezing your toes with the rest of the muscles on the bottom of the foot. If you can do this, the muscles work fine and there is no need for strengthening exercises. (These muscles may be too *tight*, as discussed below.) If you cannot perform this task, start with a few seconds of trying to pick up the sock. You should be able to lift the front of your foot off the floor while holding the sock. More than a few seconds may fatigue the muscles, so you can limit the activity to this time frame. Perform this exercise several times a day, gradually building up to about one minute for each foot. As it becomes easier, you can switch from sock or towel to a marble or small ball for a better workout.

2. Once you can more easily pick up the sock or marble, you can begin the next part of this exercise. This involves lifting the sock or marble and moving it left and right. With your heel planted firmly on the floor, pick up the sock or marble and move it as far to the left as you can, rotating on your heel. Next, move it as far to the right as you can, keeping your heel on the floor. Gradually, bring your foot (holding the sock or marble) farther and farther to the left and right each time. Be sure to keep your heel on the floor. You should feel the muscles in your leg as you perform this task. Work up

to performing this part of the exercise for about two minutes in each foot.

3. The third part of the strengthening exercises involves lifting up your foot as far as possible while holding the sock or marble. This strengthens the tibialis anterior muscle more than the previous routine. After picking up the sock or marble, lift your foot straight up, as far up as it will go. Next, bring the sock or marble as far right as possible and place it on the floor. Then do the same to the left. In all movements, raise your foot as high as possible. Over time, you'll increase your range of motion as the tibialis anterior strengthens.

Once you have strengthened your foot muscles, you can maintain your strength through normal use, so you generally don't have to continue the exercises. This is especially true if you spend time being barefoot.

Tight Muscles

In some situations, certain muscles may become too tight. This problem is most often secondary to another muscle being too weak or inhibited. In some situations, the plantar muscles and calf muscles (gastrocnemius and soleus) may be too tight. These problems are sometimes termed *plantar fasciitis* or *Achilles tendonitis*. As these names imply inflammation, which is not usually the case, I prefer not to use them. Instead, these types of problems should just be referred to as muscle imbalances.

If you have pain on the bottoms of your feet but are able to pick up a towel with your plantar muscles as discussed above, they are probably too tight. Plantar muscles that are too tight can be very painful and are most noticeable when you take your first steps out of bed in the morning–the bottoms of your feet are tight and painful but loosen up as you move around.

The problem is often secondary to other muscle inhibition, with the tibialis posterior being a common cause. If this is the case, treatment should be directed at the tibialis posterior muscle.

The best way to reduce the tightness in the plantar muscles is with a golf ball. Place a golf ball on the floor. A thin carpet or bare floor works best. Place your bare foot on top of the golf ball and roll your foot on top of the ball. Apply sufficient weight to feel the tight muscles, but not so much as to cause pain. Roll the ball as far forward as you can, and as far back as you can. Be sure to reach the whole width of the foot as well. Perform this task for two to five minutes with each foot, spending up to ten minutes total. Be aware that relief may only be symptomatic if the primary problem is not addressed.

The gastrocnemius and soleus can also become too tight due to muscle imbalance. The best and safest approach is to perform a gentle *active static stretch* to help balance the muscles. This is accomplished in the sitting position with bare feet (or socks), the knees straight, and the heels resting on the floor. *Slowly* raise the feet by bringing your toes as high up toward your head as possible. Hold this position for twenty to thirty seconds if you can, and then slowly return the feet to normal. Maintain the heels on the floor during this exercise. Perform this three to four times, but only if it does not cause pain or cramping. Doing this routine morning and evening can help reduce tightness not only in the gastrocnemius and soleus muscles, but the plantar muscles as well. You can also perform this light stretch during the day as needed for relief of symptoms.

SOFT TAPING

There are many different types of taping used by a lot of therapists for a variety of foot problems. In some cases, these are for emergency purposes, such as following an accident to provide temporary immobilization. In other cases, it's used during an athletic event. And at other times, it's to provide support during a healing process. Previously we discussed the problem associated with taping, describing how this action may weaken the muscles and ligaments. Here I discuss a different type of taping I refer to as *soft taping*.

The intention of soft taping is *not* to support the foot or ankle, but to stimulate the sensitive nerves to improve foot-sense. It is a very light taping with just two pieces of tape. Remember that foot-sense is associated with the feeling of position and movement. The loss of foot-sense can lead to dysfunction and injury, while improving this awareness can restore normal foot function.

Soft taping of the lower leg, ankle, and foot improves foot-sense and can be a powerful therapeutic tool for many types of chronic foot problems. These include recurrent sprained ankles, plantar problems, heel problems, and many others, including those annoying undiagnosed conditions.

Soft taping is accomplished with two simple steps. It requires one-inch white athletic tape available in most drug stores. Slightly wider or thinner tape is acceptable. Both pieces should be about twelve inches long, more for larger and less for smaller bodies. Here are the two steps:

■   First, place one piece of tape around the lowest part of the leg, just above the two prominent bones on either side of the ankle. This piece should overlap itself by a couple of inches, feel snug *but not tight*, and should stick to the leg.

- Second, attach another piece of tape on to the first, facing downward, and wrap it down the outside and under the midfoot. Wrap it up the inside of the ankle at the middle of the arch, and attach it to the other side of the first piece. (See Figure 11.1) If the second piece of tape does not stick well to the first, apply a short, two-inch piece over the attachments to help it stick.

The goal is not to support the foot or ankle, so you should not feel the tape providing any supporting role. It should be comfortable, not tight. At the end of the day when you may have more fluid in your foot and ankle, it still should not be tight or uncomfortable. For this reason, in some people it's best to apply the tape in the evening.

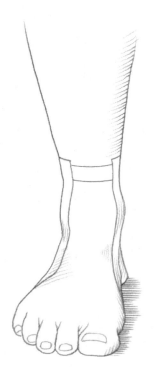

FIGURE 11.1 Soft taping.

Leave the tape on for several days. It will gradually begin to peel off. It should not be soaked in a bath but can be gotten wet from a shower and carefully dried. Remove it after a few days and leave it off for a week. If you are spending time barefoot and performing the other therapeutic routines already discussed, you should see improvement in the function of your foot after the first application. If there is no improvement or only very small improvement, tape the foot and ankle again for the same period of time.

In some situations, taping may have to be done regularly. This may be the case if you have worn bad shoes for a long time, if you have to wear heavy or oversupported shoes for work or sports, for any footwear that is not comfortable (until you buy new shoes), or as part of a rehabilitation program for a more severe problem such as a stroke or spinal injury.

Other methods of achieving improved foot-sense can be attained with an ankle board, balancing actions with eyes closed, slant-board exercises, and other exercises not detailed here. However, the activities discussed above, plus being barefoot, can provide at least equal benefits and often much more with the least amount of time, effort, and equipment.

Many people use stretching for their foot problems, the topic of the next chapter.

12

STRETCHING YOUR FOOT

If the notion of stretching your foot seems odd, the concept of stretching is equally peculiar to me and many other health professionals. Stretching as a remedy for various foot and ankle problems is common, especially in the calf muscles. But stretching is not a routine embraced by all athletes. Many of them, including a lot of professionals, don't stretch–and they are not necessarily more injured. In fact, stretching can *contribute* to injury in many cases, as there may be more injuries in both athletes and nonathletes who stretch than in those who do not.

Stretching is an individual issue. It's a complex, controversial, and inconclusive matter. Most people do not need to stretch as their natural activity provides for sufficient joint movement. Even athletes, if they participate in a proper active warm-up, usually don't truly need to stretch. Athletes who require greater-than-normal flexibility, such as dancers, and track and field participants, may need to stretch.

WHY STRETCH?

Most people stretch to increase their joint ranges of motion and consider it a way to prevent injuries. Of course, untold numbers of people spend a brief period of time first thing in the morning touching–or trying to touch–their toes thinking this somehow has some therapeutic value. In most cases, it can do more harm than good, and sound scientific evidence for the preventive effect of stretching is contradictory. Common injuries in sports occur most in the muscles that are most stretched.

The belief that a greater range of motion, also referred to as flexibility, in your joints can prevent injury is usually wrong. Studies actually demonstrate that increased flexibility produces more injuries, not fewer.

Too little flexibility can also contribute to injuries, so it's a balance that should be sought.

TYPES OF STRETCHES

Part of the controversy that surrounds stretching results from the difference between *ballistic* and *static* stretching, the two basic types. Other forms of stretching may exist, but they are variations of ballistic and static stretching.

BALLISTIC STRETCHING

- Ballistic stretching involves repetitive, bouncing movements that use the body's momentum and weight to repeatedly stretch a joint. This is the most common type of stretching performed and may be the most harmful. The reason this is so common is that most stretchers are in a hurry.
- Ballistic stretching can activate the *stretch reflex* in muscles and actually *increase* tension and the risk for small tears in the muscle.

STATIC STRETCHING

- Static stretching may be helpful for those who truly need to stretch–not the majority for sure. It involves very slowly stretching the muscle to a point when slight tension is felt, and then holding it for up to thirty seconds. Each muscle group should be carefully stretched one after the other three to four times. Obviously this takes time and discipline. Herein lies one of the problems–most people don't take the proper time to stretch this way. The result is they perform ballistic stretching. When performed properly, static stretching relaxes the muscle. However, note the substantial time commitment.
- Static stretching can be done two ways–*actively* or *passively.* Active static stretching contracts the opposite, or *antagonist,* muscles. For example, in this case contracting the tibialis anterior muscle by raising your foot and toes up as high as possible will gently and safely stretch the gastrocnemius and soleus muscles. This stretch was discussed in the last chapter.
- Passive static stretching typically requires the weight of your body or the force by another person to stretch a muscle or muscle group.

While a general stretch may help loosen a particular muscle or muscle group, it can at the same time worsen the *balance* of muscles. Recall that muscle imbalance consists of 1) a muscle that is too tight and 2) a muscle that is inhibited or too long. Stretching the inhibited muscle makes it longer and therefore reduces its function even more, creating further imbalance. For example, even when properly done, stretching the calf can relieve tightness of the gastrocnemius and soleus muscles, but worsen an already inhibited tibialis posterior muscle. The net result is more muscle imbalance that can adversely affect foot function.

WARMING UP YOUR FEET

If it's improved foot function you want, warming up your feet is the activity that will provide it. Warming up means getting more blood circulating throughout the muscles in your feet. This is usually accomplished in the course of just walking around, especially when barefoot. But if you're planning a long walk, jog, run, or any exercise including being on your feet for a longer than normal period, warm them up first by spending at least ten minutes walking around the house barefoot.

For those people who need more flexibility, *proper* stretching routines should be performed *after* warming up the feet. Rather than stretch your muscles to get better foot function, perform the activities discussed in these last two chapters and warm up your feet to obtain adequate flexibility for the activities you're doing.

Additional benefits may be obtained from hands-on techniques, the topic of the next chapter.

13

HANDS-ON TECHNIQUES

Restoring normal muscle function is a key part of successful therapy. This can be accomplished with a number of hands-on techniques that involve relatively simple treatment of muscles on specific areas of the foot using finger pressure. Improving muscle function also improves the performance of ligaments and tendons, joints and bone, and increases foot-sense.

There are various names that describe the many hands-on techniques commonly used for foot problems, including types of massage, different forms of acupuncture and acupressure, reflexology, trigger point therapy, and so forth. The majority of foot problems will respond to the therapies previously discussed, along with those described in this chapter under the general heading of massage and acupressure.

Applying these therapies should never be painful. Nor should you use any of these techniques when there is inflammation or edema. When in doubt, avoid treating the area.

When performed by a health professional, treatment of specific areas may cause a *momentary* unpleasant feeling during a massage or other treatment. A trained professional may find this is necessary to obtain the appropriate therapeutic outcome.

FOOT MASSAGE

Manual massage is perhaps the oldest hands-on remedy. Its first appearance as part of a defined therapeutic regime may have been more than five thousand years ago in Chinese medicine, which joined massage, acupuncture, manipulation, and a number of other remedies. Today it is a popular therapy performed by professional massage therapists and others. In its basic form, massage can be self-administered, although it's best when someone else does it.

Foot massage need not be done with hard pressure, and it should not be painful. Like other approaches described in this book, such as being barefoot or using a cold footbath, the apparently simple techniques are often mistaken for not being therapeutic enough. But a simple foot massage can do wonders for unhealthy feet, and feel just as good.

Massage should begin with a light, soft, gentle rubbing of the foot, much like kneading bread. A *small amount* of oil to assist with the motions of the hands on the skin may be helpful, but it is not always necessary. The best oil to use is almond oil, but extra virgin olive oil works well, too. Almond oil should be refrigerated when not in use and gently warmed under running water before use. Emu oil works well and has anti-inflammatory actions. Coconut oil also works well. None of these other oils needs refrigeration. Avoid putting anything on the skin that you would not eat since it can be easily absorbed into the body. Mineral oil, vegetable oils, or those oils with chemicals, including fragrances, can be unhealthy and are not recommended.

The massage should include all areas from the ends of the toes to the ankles and up the leg. Include gently moving the joints in all directions, but without forcing any motion. Gradually, apply more pressure, especially in areas where the muscles are larger or tighter, such as the bottoms of the feet and in the calf. In areas of extreme tenderness, such as trigger points (discussed below), specific finger pressure works best.

It's best to massage the foot when it's completely relaxed, the reason it's best when someone else is doing the work.

Improving Foot-Sense

By massaging the feet and up into the legs, improvements in foot-sense can easily and quickly be achieved. Since the lack of or reduction in foot-sense is such a common problem and is a significant contribution to other foot problems, any activity that improves foot-sense makes great sense.

As each degree of firmness is applied during the massage, a different level of foot-sense can be derived. So begin with a very light touch and progress to more firm pressure without causing pain. Many nerves that promote foot-sense are found in the joints, and moving them during massage is especially therapeutic.

Foot massage works especially well in conjunction with other therapies, including barefoot activity and soft taping.

TRIGGER POINTS

As you massage the foot muscles you will often notice small tender areas. These may be *trigger points*. A trigger point is an irritated area in the muscle that causes the muscle to become tighter or an abnormal area of the muscle that has tightened considerably. Once a trigger point is established, it can remain for a long time–months and years. This limits the function of the muscle including reduced range of motion in the joints attached to the muscle. Most importantly, the trigger point is usually associated with pain.

The pain of a trigger point is typically felt, or *referred* to a different area of the body. For example, a trigger point in the calf may cause pain in the heel, while the trigger point itself may not be painful until massaged. A trigger point usually has exquisite tenderness. Slow, sustained hand or finger pressure and rubbing can help eliminate the trigger point. Acupuncture points, discussed below, often co-exist with trigger points.

Trigger points can develop in the muscles from various insults to the body, such as a muscle injury, a sprain, a broken bone, reduced activity or immobilization, excess activity, and even stress.

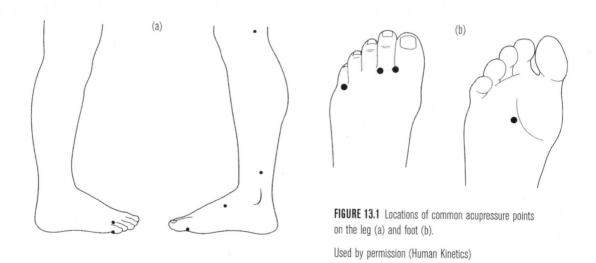

FIGURE 13.1 Locations of common acupressure points on the leg (a) and foot (b).

Used by permission (Human Kinetics)

ACUPRESSURE

Acu*puncture* and acu*pressure* are two different but common methods of treating specific points on the traditional Chinese meridians. Acupuncture uses needles to puncture the skin to provide treatment, but acupressure requires only finger pressure. I will not discuss the use of acupuncture, as acupressure can be just as effective.

Acupressure can be safe and effective without having to pierce the skin. The pressure used is not hard enough to cause pain, but even very mild pressure is sufficient in most cases to obtain good results.

There are hundreds of acupressure points all over the body, but only a small number of very important points on the feet and legs. Some points on the face are used for pain control for the feet; these are discussed in the next chapter.

There are two approaches to using acupressure points. First, all the key points in the foot and leg can be treated. See Figures 13.1, a and b. Second, only one or two of the most important key points can be treated. For example, after a thorough evaluation a professional may find one or two points that need treatment. In most cases, this is difficult to determine without additional training.

The easiest way to treat these acupressure points is to apply mild to moderate pressure on the point with the tip of your finger. Those points that require treatment will be the most tender. They should not cause significant pain, but they may be very sore in some cases. Rub the point for about ten to twenty seconds. If it is tender, this treatment should reduce the tenderness. If it does not, the point may be a trigger point that needs longer stimulation to eliminate the tenderness.

Other acupressure points are very useful to control pain, which we'll discuss in the next chapter.

1 4

PAIN CONTROL

This chapter focuses on a relatively simple technique for pain control that utilizes the Chinese meridian system. Similar therapies were introduced in the last chapter to improve muscle function. The points used for pain control here are in a different location–specifically on the face. Despite the fact that the foot is at the other end of the body from the face, treating these points as opposed to others used for pain control has proved most effective.

This chapter also discusses some natural methods of pain control and reviews how certain drugs affect pain.

Pain can be a very important symptom, despite its discomfort and frequent disability. Pain offers benefits that help you find the problem, recover more quickly, and prevent further damage:

- Pain informs you there is a problem. In many cases, pain is the only symptom informing you a problem exists. Without pain, the problem could worsen beyond the point of the body's ability to recover.
- Pain helps your body compensate by shifting weight bearing away from the problem area. Without compensation, normal standing, for example, could further worsen both pain and the area of injury.
- Pain usually prevents you from using the problem area, which can further damage an injury. Our "no pain no gain" society tends to counter common sense, and many people try to ignore pain or cover it up with painkillers.
- Pain patterns can help health care professionals assess the source of the problem.

Through *natural* pain control techniques, there is virtually no risk of covering up pain too much and thus removing pain's potential benefits. While natural pain control techniques are very effective and can significantly reduce or even eliminate pain, it is not like being sedated by drugs, which can not only completely eliminate pain but also the body's awareness of it. If pain is completely eliminated our body can forget there is still a problem, will no longer compensate for it, and we may use the area of injury excessively when what it really needs is rest.

The *lack* of pain is also an important consideration. The lack of pain does not mean there is not a problem, as many types of dysfunction exist without pain.

Remember, pain is not just a mechanical problem, but a chemical one as well. And, pain is an emotion.

NATURAL PAIN CONTROL

The evolution of our body has provided us with natural pain control mechanisms. These come in two forms: touching and diet.

TOUCHING

When the average person injuries a foot, the first thing he or she does instinctively is to reach down and lightly rub the area of pain. This is the oldest form of pain control and one used not only by humans but other animals as well (more often by licking).

Gently rubbing the skin at or near the area of pain and/or injury stimulates local nerve endings that have the effect of reducing the pain. Similar mechanisms are used to control pain through electrical stimulation and acupuncture. The results using this method may not be long lasting, but you can gently rub areas of pain every hour if necessary.

DIET

Many are surprised to learn that diet can influence pain tolerance. This is related to changes in the body's production of pain chemicals, inflammation, and the brain's response to eating certain types of foods.

Certain dietary fats can help reduce chronic pain. The most effective are the omega-3 fats–called EPA–found in fish oil. These fats reduce certain chemicals that cause inflammation and pain. Vegetable-source omega-3 fats, such as flax oil, are much less effective. Olive oil, too, may help reduce pain.

Other dietary fats can promote pain. These include trans fats, found in hydrogenated and partially hydrogenated oils; high intakes of saturated fats, especially from dairy; and high intakes from most vegetable oils. Fats influence pain by increasing or decreasing inflammation.

Foods high in sugars, starches, and other refined carbohydrates, such as sweets, soda, fruit juice, and white flour products like bagels, muffins, chips, cereals, and so forth, can *increase* pain by increasing inflammation and by changing brain chemistry.

Certain stimulants such as caffeine may not increase pain directly, but can increase your *awareness* of pain. The same is true during periods of high anxiety. Reducing caffeine, and anxiety, may be helpful to ease pain.

Food allergies can increase pain because of increased production of histamine by the body. Histamine can increase pain directly. Environmental allergies, such as pollen, can also increase histamine and cause pain.

The relationship between food and foot health is discussed in more detail in the next chapter.

CHEMICAL PAIN CONTROL

In addition to dietary factors that change the chemistry of the body, the most commonly used method of controlling pain is with non-steroidal anti-inflammatory drugs (NSAIDs), including aspirin. This is, perhaps, the most commonly used class of drugs worldwide. As the name implies, aspirin and other NSAIDs have anti-inflammatory effects. Not only is inflammation a common cause of pain, but the same chemicals produced in the body that cause inflammation can also cause pain.

Other drugs, the most common being acetaminophen (Tylenol, Anacin, Excedrin, etc.) have analgesic effects, meaning they "numb" pain through mechanisms other than controlling inflammation. Tranquilizers can reduce pain by reducing anxiety, and alcohol can suppress pain through sedation, although small amounts may amplify pain.

The potential problem with many drugs is their significant side effects. NSAIDs may be the most significant (we're all aware of the effects of excess alcohol use). NSAIDs are commonly associated with an increased incidence of stomach and duodenal ulcers and intestinal bleeding. Virtually everyone who takes aspirin, for example, has some intestinal bleeding. The use of NSAIDs can produce muscle dysfunction, can adversely affect cartilage repair around the joints, and can even impair healing of a bone fracture and other injuries. They can cause kidney damage, especially in those who are dehydrated, a common occurrence in those who exercise. Other potential side effects of NSAIDs include headaches, skin rash, ringing in the ears (tinnitus), and drowsiness. Reye's syndrome is a potentially fatal condition in children that has been associated with use of aspirin products taken during viral infections.

Statistics show that complications arising from NSAID use contribute to 16,500 deaths and 103,000 hospitalizations yearly. Acetaminophen overdose is not uncommon, but even "normal" use puts significant stress on the liver, the site of drug elimination. In addition, most of these pain medicines can interfere with normal sleep patterns, including suppression of melatonin, an important hormone associated with proper sleep and other healthy functions.

PAIN CONTROL POINTS

Before relying on drugs to treat common pain problems, consider a natural remedy. A variety of meridian points can be successfully used for pain control. During my twenty years in private practice, I used these points regularly for pain control, and with great success. But I always sought to find and correct the cause of the pain—something you must also resolve.

This section discusses the most effective points for controlling pain in the feet, ankles, and lower legs. These points are all located on the face. In traditional Chinese medicine they are called the *beginning* and *end* points because they are the start or end of certain acupuncture meridians.

FINDING THE RIGHT POINT

Certain areas on the feet, ankles, and legs correspond with one of three pairs of points on the face—one of six points total. Figures 14.1a and 14.1b show the areas on the feet, ankles, and legs that correspond to the same numbered point on the face shown in Figure 14.1c. Three examples are given here.

- ■ *Example 1:* If you have pain from stubbing your right big toe, this is located in area 1. This corresponds to point number 1 on the face. This point is located on the right side of the face, on the bone just outside the eye (see Figure 14.1c). Tap this point approximately one hundred times to reduce pain in the big toe.
- ■ *Example 2:* If you have pain in your left heel, this is located in area 3 and the corresponding point on the face is number 3. This point is located on the upper part of the inside portion of your nose on the left, just inside to the inner corner of the eye (see Figure 14.1c). Tap this point approximately one hundred times to reduce heel pain.
- ■ *Example 3:* If you have pain on top of the middle right foot, this is located in area 2 and the corresponding point on the face is number 2. This point is located just under the middle of the right

eye on the check bone (see Figure 14.1c). Tap this point approximately one hundred times to reduce pain on this area of the ankle.

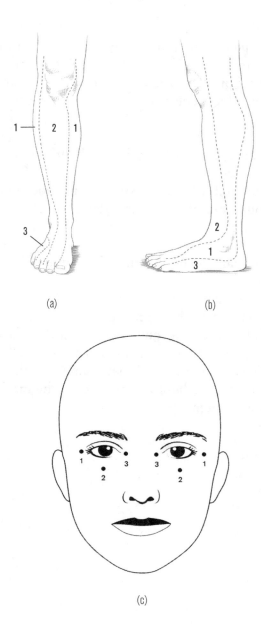

FIGURE 14.1 Pain control. Choose the area of pain (a and b) and treat the corresponding point on the face. (c) (Note: back of legs and bottoms of feet is number 3.)

Used by permission (Human Kinetics)

(a)   (b)

(c)

The points tapped on the face should be on the same side of the body as the pain. So if you stub your right toe, you will treat point number 1 on the right side.

Much of this information is adapted from traditional Chinese medicine and from Dr. Walter H. Schmitt's booklet *Stop Your Pain Now!*

(Innovations in Healthcare Group LLC, 20102 Spring Meadow Drive, Chapel Hill, North Carolina 27514).

TREATING THE POINTS

You can treat the points on your face by tapping them with the tips of your finger with mild to moderate pressure. Tap relatively fast, about two taps per second or faster, for approximately one hundred taps.

To improve the effectiveness of this technique, perform the following *while* tapping:

- Move the area of pain (if possible) or lightly touch the area with your other hand.
- Think about and focus on the pain and its location.
- Think about when the pain first started (such as an accident or specific incident).

This will help the brain be more aware of the area of pain and help reduce the pain more.

The points can be tapped several times a day if necessary. Occasionally, it may take more than a hundred taps, and at other times fewer taps will be effective. If more than one area on the foot, ankle, or leg is painful, you can tap more than one point. It's not unusual to reduce pain significantly or even completely eliminate pain using this technique.

Many factors that contribute to pain are biochemical, which we'll discuss in the next chapter.

15

BIOCHEMICAL FOOT FACTORS

In addition to physical balance problems in the foot's structure, situations such as inflammation, poor circulation, and infections may be present and reflect imbalance in the body's natural chemistry, called biochemistry. In the majority of cases diet, dietary supplements, and exercise can correct these chemical imbalances. In some cases a health care professional may be needed, as discussed in Chapter 17.

CHRONIC INFLAMMATION

Inflammation is typically thought of as a swollen, painful, or otherwise uncomfortable area of the body. It's common in a joint from arthritis, for example, or the result of stubbing your toe. For most people, inflammation occurs without any symptoms. Initially, inflammation is the protective reaction by the body, responding to some physical or chemical injury. Long-term inflammation is more serious.

TWO TYPES OF INFLAMMATION

Acute inflammation is a normal response by the body and is typically accompanied by pain, swelling, redness, and heat. Without this normal inflammation, we would not recover from a day at the office, a workout, or a walk to the mailbox. There are three important functions of normal inflammation: First, inflammation is the initial step in the healing or repair process after some physical or chemical injury or stress, no matter how minor. Without it, even a minor stubbed toe could worsen and result in a serious problem. Second, inflammation prevents the spread of damaged cells to other areas of the body that could cause secondary problems. A local toenail infection, for example, can be contained due to the inflammatory response, instead of causing a bodywide infection. And third, inflammation rids the body of damaged and dead cells. This very important task is more than just an act of housecleaning.

Normally, the inflammatory–anti-inflammatory cycle is somewhat like an "on-off" switch: Inflammation is turned on when needed for healing and repair (by the body's natural inflammatory chemicals), and then turned off when not needed (by our natural anti-inflammatory chemicals).

Chronic inflammation is an abnormal condition of long-term inflammation. It can cause or is associated with ill health and disease. Uncontrolled acute inflammation can lead to chronic inflammation. This transition may take place due to continued physical or chemical stress. Examples include local trauma such as jamming the toes in your shoes, infection, or poor diet. Many foot problems are associated with chronic inflammation, from arthritis to plantar fasciitis to Achilles tendonitis. Any word ending in "itis" refers to inflammation.

Chronic inflammation is typically the first stage of many more serious conditions, not only in the feet but also throughout the body. These include ulcers, poor circulation, vascular disease, heart disease, and cancer.

Chronic inflammation can develop from biochemical imbalance from the wrong dietary fats, inadequate nutrient intake, and dietary factors that block anti-inflammatory chemicals. Any of these common causes of chronic inflammation could seriously affect our feet. By balancing dietary fats, we can eliminate chronic inflammation.

Many natural inflammatory and anti-inflammatory chemicals are heavily influenced by diet. Two key items that can have a dramatic effect on reducing unwanted inflammation in the body are discussed below:

1. Balance dietary fats.
2. Make sure you have all the nutrients to maintain the balanced fats.

THE ABCS OF FAT

The fats in our diet play a vital role in the inflammatory–anti-inflammatory cycle–where inflammation is created to heal and recover a certain area, followed by the production of anti-inflammatory chemicals when the healing is completed. Three fats, labeled as A, B, and C for convenience, are important to keep balanced if you're going to control inflammation.

- *A fats:* These include most vegetable oils that contain a high level of omega-6 polyunsaturated oils such as corn, safflower, sunflower, peanut, cottonseed, sesame, and soy oils.
- *B fats:* These are mostly made up of saturated fats, especially those found in dairy products such as milk, butter, cheese, and cream. Lesser amounts are found in meats, egg yolks, and shellfish.
- *C fats:* These include omega-3 polyunsaturated oils found mostly in certain cold-water fish such as salmon, mackerel, and sardines, and small amounts can also be found in flax, walnuts, pumpkin seeds, and beans.

These three groups of fats are converted in the body to natural chemicals that are either inflammatory or anti-inflammatory. Most of these are called *eicosanoids* (pronounced i-COS-an-oids). These chemicals have very powerful physiological effects: A and C fats have anti-inflammatory effects and the B fats have inflammatory effects. See table below.

TABLE 15.1 The ABCs of fats.

Fats:	A	B	C
	↓	↓	↓
Effects:	anti-inflammatory	inflammatory	anti-inflammatory

A key concern is that some A fats can be converted to B fats along the way. This happens when there are too many A fats in the diet. It means that potentially, many A fats, although polyunsaturated, will eventually turn into inflammatory chemicals rather than anti-inflammatory ones. In essence, they function just like saturated fats. When this happens, it's as if you are eating too many B fats. See table below.

TABLE 15.2 A fats can convert to B fats.

A fats	B fats	C fats
↓	↓	↓
→	→	→
↓	↓	↓
anti-inflammatory	inflammatory	anti-inflammatory

This problem can be prevented by reducing your intake of A fats so that they're balanced with the B and C fats. In addition, raw sesame seed oil is the best A fat to use regularly because it contains a natural substance called *sesamin* that helps prevent A fats from converting to B fats. Fish oil also helps prevent A fats from converting to B fats.

Balancing dietary fats is best accomplished by eating approximately equal amounts of A, B, and C fats. It's not necessary to do this at each and every meal, but over the course of a day and/or week is fine.

Scientists tell us that the diets of early humans had an optimal balance of fats, with similar amounts of omega-6 and omega-3 fats consumed. Today, however, people commonly eat five, ten, or often twenty times the amount of omega-6 fats—a problem that can lead to chronic inflammation.

One way of adjusting your diet is to use monounsaturated fats in place of all omega-6 fats in food preparation. These are omega-9 fats and they are neither A, B, nor C. This will reduce your intake of A fats, and monounsaturated oils can also help reduce inflammation. High monounsaturated oils include extra virgin olive, almond, and walnut. Avocados are also an excellent food high in these healthy fats.

It should be noted that most foods contain a mixture of A, B, and C fats, but the dominant forms are contained in those described above.

NUTRIENTS TO MAINTAIN FAT BALANCE

Conversion of A and C fats to anti-inflammatory chemicals requires a number of important nutrients. It's important to obtain these through your diet. A list of these nutrients and food sources are listed below:

Nutrient	Food Sources
Vitamin B6	fish, eggs, brown rice, oats, beans, avocado, walnuts
Niacin	meats, eggs, nuts, seeds
Vitamin E	raw green leafy vegetables, raw nuts
Vitamin C	fresh vegetables and fruits
Magnesium	green vegetables, nuts, seeds, legumes
Zinc	meats, eggs, seafood

SUPPLEMENTS

Because we don't eat as much cold-water fish as did our ancestors, and our diets contain unusually high levels of A fats from vegetable oils, it's difficult to balance our fats without supplementing our diet. Fish oil capsules (not fish *liver* oil) can accomplish this because of their high amounts of EPA—one of the important fats with powerful anti-inflammatory effects. For many people, beginning with one to three capsules taken three times daily is a good start; more for others with various foot problems caused by arthritis or diabetic ulcers, for example, or for those recovering from foot surgery. For those who have exceptionally good diets, one or two capsules per day may be sufficient.

When eating fish avoid overcooking it, as too much heat will destroy the omega-3 fats. Raw fish, common in Japanese restaurants (called *sashimi*), is ideal. Farmed fish contains much less or no omega-3 fat.

Many fish oil products sold today may be contaminated with toxic metals found in many ocean fish. To ensure this is not the case, make sure the product states that it has been tested for potential contamination. A good indication the product is toxic-free is that it's also free of cholesterol, as stated on the label (when the toxic chemicals are removed, so goes the cholesterol).

FOODS AND INFLAMMATION

Other natural foods have powerful anti-inflammatory actions. These include ginger, turmeric, onions, garlic, and citrus peel.

Foods that promote inflammation include trans fat found in hydrogenated and partially hydrogenated oils. These fats block the production of anti-inflammatory chemicals. The most popular food containing these fats is margarine. Excess alcohol can also promote inflammation, while moderate levels can be anti-inflammatory. Sugar and other sweet foods, and refined flour products as noted above can also increase inflammation.

NSAIDs reduce inflammation by inhibiting the conversion of B fats to inflammatory chemicals. Unfortunately, they also inhibit natural anti-inflammatory chemicals, too, so the body never really balances itself. NSAIDs, including their side effects, were discussed in the previous chapter.

POOR CIRCULATION

There are two issues regarding circulation that are important in maintaining healthy feet throughout life. We have already discussed the first—avoiding chronic inflammation and if you have it, correcting it. The second is physical activity.

Through physical activity our muscles work harder than when they are at rest. This movement forces more blood through the blood vessels that feed the muscles oxygen and other nutrients. These nutrients not only benefit the muscles but all areas of the feet–from the skin down to the innermost area of bone. This allows our feet to recover from day-to-day activity, build new cells, and maintain optimal function.

On one hand, it's very simple–we need to be active on a regular basis to have healthy feet. But it's not always that easy. Our society makes it difficult with the many conveniences that keep us inactive. And the problem is worsening as our next generation–our children–have become the most inactive and out of shape in the history of the human race. Computer games, TV, inactive parents, and other negative factors all contribute.

One result of inactivity is poor circulation. Toes and other areas of the foot become susceptible to ill health, poor function, and, potentially, disease.

EASY EXERCISE

Without natural activity, such as performing large amounts of manual work every day, our only other option is exercise. For many people, just the thought of exercise is tiring. One reason is our "no pain no gain" approach, which proposes that we have to work out real hard to get benefits. It conjures up images of sweaty gyms with sculpted bodies. But in reality, this is not necessary to accomplish a lifetime of healthy feet.

What's most important to improve the health of your feet, especially in terms of circulation, is easy aerobic exercise. Easy to the point where when you're done, you almost feel as if you've not done anything, and could do it all over again. For many people, this translates to thirty minutes of easy walking a day. If you are a beginner, start with five, ten, or fifteen minutes a day if that's easier. Slowly working your way up to thirty minutes will be enjoyable. Add more time if you like, but do it slowly as you build up your fitness.

It's not necessary to exercise every day. Five days a week is very effective, six if you're so inclined. Four days a week may only keep you from getting more out of shape. It's also not necessary to walk. You can swim, ride a bike, dance, or perform a variety of easy activities, even alternate through the week. I'd suggest avoiding hard or potentially hard activity like jogging or running unless you're starting in better shape, and carefully monitor your heart rate. Walking and other weight-bearing workouts have the added benefits of gravity, which further helps strengthen bones.

INFECTIONS, ULCERS, AND SKIN REACTIONS

A discussion about foot infections, ulcers, and adverse skin reactions is important, although these problems are much less common than others described in this book. But if you have them, they're very important, and addressing them should be a primary concern.

Foot infections are the most common of this group, especially fungal infections. Ulcers occur in those who are diabetic or are immobile (such as those who require prolonged bed rest), and adverse reactions sometimes occur due to chemical sensitivity, such as to rubber or latex materials in shoes or clothing.

In most if not all of these problems, there is an underlying chronic inflammation present. In addition, in most cases circulation is poor. By addressing these two topics, a person often reduces or eliminates many common infections, ulcers, and other adverse reactions and can prevent them as well. Incidentally, those who wear shoes all the time are much more susceptible to fungal infections.

A discussion about serious infections or ulcers goes beyond the scope of this book and should be discussed with your doctor. This section will address some of the more common problems you can treat with home remedies while working with your doctor.

INFECTIONS

Bacterial infections are usually more serious than fungal infections, which are quite common. Bacterial infections may be systemic (a bodywide infection) or local, such as an ingrown toenail that has become infected. Your doctor should treat bacterial infections.

Fungal infections are common, especially in those who wear shoes all the time. Regular shoe wear creates a perfect environment for fungal growth—warm and moist. It's quite possible that most people, if not everyone, has a fungus on or in their feet. If the environment you create for your feet is right for the fungus to grow, you will have a problem. But if you allow your feet to dry completely after bathing—by remaining barefoot for sufficient time to allow the feet to thoroughly dry—you will be much less likely to allow fungal growth. This is especially true during the warmer months, when your feet don't dry as easily, but also in cooler environments when your feet are covered most of the time.

Fungal infections are first noticed when the skin between the toes gets itchy and cracks. In more chronic infections, the nails are adversely affected and can be very uncomfortable or even painful. This is especially common in those with diabetes or weakened immune systems.

Simple fungal infections may be successfully treated by allowing the feet to completely dry following any activity that moistens them, including bathing, exercise, or even a day in shoes or boots. In this case, removing the socks as well is important to obtain complete drying. This could take an hour or more in a relatively dry environment, longer when it's more humid. This is by far the most important factor to reduce and prevent foot infections.

A number of other habits are very helpful to reduce and prevent foot infections:

- Rinse your feet every day, and if you have chronic infections, scrub your feet with a washcloth or brush. Use only plain soap without fragrance or other chemicals, and only when your feet require a more thorough cleaning.
- Thoroughly dry your feet. This means sitting down and making it a point to dry all areas of the feet, especially in between the toes and the nails. If necessary, use a hairdryer briefly, on a low setting.
- Be sure the insides and outsides of your shoes are dry before wearing them.
- Clean the insides of your shoes, especially if they get damp. Some sports shoes can be put in the washing machine.
- Be sure your socks are completely dry before wearing them.
- Change your socks daily.

Various natural topical remedies can be very effective for fungal infections. These include eucalyptus oil, camphor, and menthol. These ingredients are also found in popular chest rubs. Over-the-counter fungal ointments can be useful, with Lamisil AT perhaps being the most effective drug. But this and other drugs can also have side effects. Be sure to read the fine print on the product packaging. Regardless of the remedy you choose, without changing the foot environment the infection will eventually return.

Treatment of more serious nail infections may require more intense care by your doctor. But it's still important to address the environment of your feet. The common drug prescribed for serious fungal infections is oral terbinafine, but before recommending it your doctor should perform a culture to confirm the diagnosis. Terbinafine is not without side effects and certain lifestyle changes may be necessary, such as avoiding alcohol. Your doctor may also want to periodically perform a blood test to make sure the drug does not adversely affect your liver.

Feet that have foul odor are usually infested with some type of microorganism, most often bacterial. These bacteria produce substances called fatty acids that have the foul odor. Follow the remedies discussed above to reduce and prevent bacterial buildup on the feet. The skin normally has natural and helpful bacteria on it at all times. Overuse of soaps, chemical powders, and antibacterial products can eliminate these

friendly bacteria, allowing other more harmful and often odor-produc-
ing bacteria to take over.

Skin Ulcers

Foot ulcers are most common in those individuals with diabetes. The vast
majority of those with diabetes have at least one foot problem because of
poor circulation, poor nervous system function, and poor wound healing
due to reduced immunity. Foot problems are the most common reason
for hospital admissions in patients with diabetes. In many cases, this is
due to not addressing many other health needs. A discussion of the foot
needs of those with diabetes or ulcers goes beyond the scope of this book.
It is strongly recommended that you discuss adequate dietary and other
requirements with your health care practitioner.

A skin ulcer is an area on the skin that has worn away due to trauma,
pressure, infection, or other causes. In addition to diabetes, other factors
that promote foot, ankle, and leg ulcers are bed rest and other inactivity such as restriction to a wheelchair or wearing a cast for a prolonged
amount of time.

Foot ulcers often lead to infections, although sometimes infections
are a cause of an ulcer. The combination of ulceration and infection
makes these problems difficult to treat. In some cases, amputation may
be necessary.

Chronic inflammation, which may occur early in the development
of diabetes, is a precursor to a foot ulcer.

Skin Reactions

A variety of skin reactions can occur in the foot, ankle, and leg usually
due to contact with certain materials in the shoes, socks, or other items
such as supports. Latex products, the most common offending substance, are manufactured from the rubber tree, with several chemicals
added during processing. These chemicals are often the cause of skin reactions. Some proteins in latex can also cause a range of mild to severe
allergic reactions.

Rubber materials and expandable elastic in shoes, socks, and supports
are the most common materials that could affect the feet, ankles, and
legs. Up to 12 percent or more of the population may be sensitive to
these products. The three most common skin reactions are discussed
here. Of the three, the most common skin reaction is *irritant contact
dermatitis*. This causes dry, itchy, irritated areas on the skin. This is not
a true allergy, but a simple local irritation of the skin.

Allergic contact dermatitis (also called *chemical sensitivity dermatitis*) is another reaction, and it usually has a delayed response. This can

cause skin reactions that may look similar to poison ivy. The rash usually begins twenty-four to forty-eight hours after contact with the offending material and may progress to oozing skin blisters or spread away from the area of skin touched by the latex.

Another reaction is a *latex allergy,* which is an *immediate hypersensitivity* that can be much more serious. Exposures to even very small amounts in susceptible individuals can trigger bodywide allergic reactions. These reactions usually begin within minutes of exposure to latex, but they can also occur hours later and can produce various symptoms. Mild reactions to latex involve skin redness, hives, or itching. More severe reactions may involve respiratory symptoms such as runny nose, sneezing, itchy eyes, scratchy throat, and asthma (difficult breathing, coughing spells, and wheezing). Rarely, shock may occur. These reactions are similar to those seen in some allergic persons following a bee sting.

Other reactions can occur due to contact with chemical residues in dyes, soaps, cosmetics, powders, or other toiletries used on the feet or in socks, stocking, or shoes. All these reactions will disappear once the offending chemical is removed.

Children are most vulnerable to chemical stresses. The proper care of children's feet is an opportunity to prevent most foot problems, as you'll learn in the next chapter.

1 6

THE EARLIEST FEET

Brimming with powerful nerve endings, a baby's feet are an opportunity to stimulate healthy neurological and physical development from the earliest age. Easy massage or even just simple regular rubbing of the feet can have potent therapeutic actions. Children of any age can benefit this way to prevent future problems. This chapter discusses some of the important aspects of children's feet and things to do to prevent the many problems associated with lifestyle problems in childhood that effect the feet in adulthood.

Preventive strategies are best implemented early in life—in this case, taking advantage of the easily accessible and effective ways to improve health through stimulation of the bottoms of the baby's feet. Foot massage at any age is therapeutic, but it is especially so in children. Regular easy rubbing of the feet, with attention to the soles, is important and enjoyed by children. This can be done daily, and especially any time a child gets bumped and bruised anywhere on their body through their daily learning experiences. (See Chapter 13 for a more detailed description of the benefits and methods of giving a massage.)

CHILDREN'S NORMAL FEET

Children most often have normal feet but they don't always look like adult feet. As children start walking, they may even appear flatfooted. This is due to the baby fat that is not only in their face and belly, but in the arches of their feet, too. This *physiologic flatfoot* appearance should not be confused with a *pathologic flatfoot* condition. Professionals, shoe companies, and others perpetuate many myths about this phenomenon.

A pathologic flatfoot condition is one where the foot and ankle are very rigid and usually requires some type of treatment. But this is rare. Many children have physiologic flatfoot, which is normal for them, and eventually they form what is known as a "normal" healthy arch. Unfortunately, too many children with physiologic flatfeet are treated for abnormal conditions, often with supports, bracing, or special shoes. This can not only be ineffective but, as studies show, puts significant psychological stress on the child, especially those who attend school. This stress can even carry over to psychological problems in adulthood.

If your health care professional recommends some type of therapy for your child's foot, consider getting one or more additional opinions.

SHOE STRESS

Earlier in this book we discussed the many potential problems associated with wearing shoes. The greatest potential risk from wearing shoes occurs in childhood. Most pathologic foot problems in children and adults are associated with early shoe wear. Studies show that young children who wear shoes earliest and longest generally have the most problems as older children and adults. This is because wearing shoes in childhood can be detrimental to normal foot development.

As a consultant for the Institutes for the Achievement of Human Potential in Philadelphia, Pennsylvania, I helped implement a barefoot strategy. Here, where well children and many types of brain-injured children are evaluated, programs used for physical, intellectual, and physiological development are most often prescribed with the recommendation that children be barefoot. This not only removes potential stress during physical movement, but also creates a positive neurological effect throughout the body.

Without shoes, children, like adults, are more stable on their feet. As such, their physical development is better and their risk of fall lessened. The incidence of falls in children, as studies show, is significantly greater with shoes than without.

As young children begin to walk, they will want to venture out into the world. In many areas they will need protection for their feet, in the form of shoes. The best shoes for children are not unlike those for adults, and, like adult shoes, their purpose is merely protective. Consider the following factors when buying shoes for children. They should:

- not "treat" or support the foot with inserts, orthotics, or other supports
- not interfere with normal movement

- be "low-top" rather than "high-top" in structure
- fit perfectly
- be very comfortable
- have a thin, rubber sole
- have a rough rather than smooth sole surface

Once children return to a safer environment, their shoes should come off.

Since shoes also alter the walking and running gait, this can be a significant source of structural stress in growing children. Consider how trees grow when blocked by other trees or subjected to other physical restraints—as they get bigger they become crooked, weaker, and more vulnerable to breaks.

COSTS

Parents are usually grateful to hear that very inexpensive shoes are quite adequate for children of any age, especially considering how many different pairs will be needed throughout childhood.

But as children become indoctrinated by TV and other sources of advertising, and see older children and athletes wearing fancy $100-plus shoes, they will want a pair. How parents manage this is very individual. But if a child is old enough to get an allowance or even work, he or she should contribute financially to expensive shoes that serve no purpose but to impress other children.

SPORTS

About thirty million children participate in sports. Unfortunately, injuries are common. More than a third of all school-aged children sustain injuries severe enough to warrant a visit to a health care practitioner. Most important is the fact that the ankle (along with the knee) is the most common area of injury in children. Most of the knee injuries are nontraumatic, meaning they are secondary. In my years of practice, most children with nontraumatic knee pain had foot problems, sometimes asymptomatic, that caused the knee problem.

Most of the injuries in children can be prevented. Many, if not most, are related to footwear. In addition to the information in this chapter, earlier chapters provided information about physical activity that can be applied to children.

Preventing foot problems in adults begins in childhood. Spending as much time barefoot is the first step to healthy feet throughout childhood and as adults.

17

FINDING A HEALTH
CARE PROFESSIONAL

There are times when the right health care professional must play a role in fixing your feet. This may include a podiatrist, applied kinesiologist, massage therapist, surgeon, or other professional. There are a number of issues to consider when searching for the right professional.

Chapter 4 outlined three therapeutic options when a foot problem develops: leave things alone and let your body correct it, help your body with some conservative remedies, or seek professional help. The decision to see certain health professionals is based on a number of factors, including type of problem, your personal beliefs and philosophy about certain practitioners, and, unfortunately, insurance coverage.

Finding a health professional who matches your particular needs is your goal. This includes finding a professional who takes adequate time during your visit, is thorough in his or her assessment, is willing and able to communicate with other professionals you currently or previously saw, and practices what he or she preaches. Unfortunately, this may take time and visits to more than just one professional. It is my strong belief that health care professionals are also teachers: The word "doctor" means teacher. So not only should you get the necessary care, but your health care professional should also explain the problems and teach you how to prevent future problems. Once you find the right match, you won't let insurance companies, distance, or other factors interfere with your relationship. The right professional won't be needed on such a regular basis in almost all cases.

TYPES OF HEALTH CARE PROFESSIONALS

For your feet, there are a number of different health care professionals who may be of service. In general, these include, from the most conservative to the more radical, massage therapists, applied kinesiologists, chiropractors, osteopaths, podiatrists, medical doctors, and surgeons. While these are the main categories of practitioners in the United States, and the ones described in this book, there may be others who can also correct foot problems.

There are two general areas of health care—often described as *complementary* and *medical.* Complementary care, sometimes referred to as *alternative,* consists of therapies outside the modern medical model of care. These may include manipulation, acupuncture, diet/nutrition, and others. Massage therapists, applied kinesiologists, chiropractors, and others are in this category. Medical care is the popular approach of hospitals and medical clinics and may include podiatrists, osteopaths, and medical doctors, with some of these professionals performing surgery.

Some individual practitioners may incorporate remedies not typically part of their profession. For example, a podiatrist may perform surgery and recommend nutritional items to speed healing. A medical doctor may use applied kinesiology and prescribe drugs, if needed. Or a massage therapist may help with your diet.

Following is a very general description of specific specialties. Be aware that individual practitioners, as noted above, may incorporate many different therapies based on interest and scope of license.

Massage Therapy

The profession of massage therapy, sometimes called therapeutic massage, comprises trained, licensed practitioners who provide various types of massage techniques. Massage therapy is sometimes recommended by both mainstream and complementary practitioners to supplement their own therapies. Massage focuses on increasing blood circulation and lymph flow, reducing muscle tension and spasm, improving joint range of motion, and helping to reduce pain. It involves soft tissue manipulation to help balance muscles and aid in stress reduction.

A variety of techniques are used in massage, including different types of Swedish massage. These help create a balancing of muscles, reductions of trigger points, and reduced muscle tightness and spasms. Massage therapists can perform treatments for specific injuries and provide regular maintenance care.

Physical Therapy

Physical therapists (PTs or physiotherapists) help restore function, improve mobility, relieve pain, and prevent or limit permanent physical disabilities of patients with various injuries or diseases. PTs must also be trained and licensed to practice. Their treatments often include exercise for patients who have been immobilized and lack flexibility, strength, or endurance.

Physical therapists may use electrical stimulation, hot packs or cold compresses, and ultrasound to relieve pain and reduce swelling. They may use traction or deep-tissue massage to relieve pain. Therapists also teach patients to use assistive devices such as crutches, prostheses, and wheelchairs. They also may show patients exercises to do at home to expedite their recovery.

Applied Kinesiology

Applied kinesiology (AK) combines many existing therapies into one system, much like Chinese medicine. Those who practice AK use manual muscle testing extensively to help determine the existence of muscle imbalance. One goal of the practitioner is to find the therapies that best match the patient's specific needs. This may include manipulation, acupuncture or acupressure, nutrition, and others. Most AK doctors also incorporate lifestyle recommendations such as exercise, diet, and stress management.

There is not a specific academic degree for AK. Rather, it is practiced by interested individuals who already possess a license to practice in another field and have taken extensive course work in AK. Applied kinesiology is utilized worldwide mostly by chiropractors, medical doctors, and osteopaths, along with a variety of other practitioners.

Chiropractic

While manipulation of the spine has been used for centuries, the chiropractic profession, which specializes in this technique, dates back to 1895. Chiropractors believe that spinal vertebra misalignments, called chiropractic subluxations, interfere with the normal activity of the nervous system to cause various functional problems. A chiropractic subluxation refers to a joint that is dysfunctional within its normal range of motion. This joint dysfunction may not necessarily cause pain, but will usually have some adverse effect elsewhere in the body, such as in the feet.

Some chiropractors also address imbalances associated with other joints, especially the feet. In the United States, chiropractors must receive a doctoral degree (a doctor of chiropractic, or D.C.) in a rigorous education nearly identical to that of medical school, except that it does not include studies in surgery. Some chiropractors are also trained in other complementary disciplines, including diet and nutrition, applied kinesiology, and Chinese medicine.

OSTEOPATHY

Traditional osteopathy is a manipulative-based therapy using a conservative nondrug approach. There is a stronger focus on the bones of the head and neck and the muscles and bones throughout the body. Some osteopaths utilize other therapies including acupuncture, diet and nutrition, and applied kinesiology. Andrew Taylor Still developed osteopathy in the 1890s, but by the 1950s the majority of osteopaths were incorporated into mainstream medicine, with some performing surgery.

Today, most osteopaths in the United States practice like medical doctors, having abandoned their traditional techniques. The doctor of osteopathy degree (D.O.) is virtually identical to a medical degree. In many parts of the world, especially in Europe, many osteopaths have maintained their traditional roles, often utilizing many complementary approaches including cranial-sacral techniques to treat problems throughout the body.

PODIATRY

Most podiatrists work exclusively with the medical or surgical needs of the foot, ankle, and lower leg. Their doctor of podiatric medicine (D.P.M.) degree is similar to a medical degree. Many podiatrists focus on specific areas such as surgery or diabetic foot care, while others have a very broad practice and may utilize various conservative therapies. As such, podiatrists treat a wide range of problems from corns, calluses, and muscle disorders to more serious injuries, infections, and surgical care for bunions and other problems.

MEDICAL DOCTORS

Medical doctors (M.D.s) usually play the role of the family doctor and may be the first to see patients with foot problems. In some cases, the M.D. will treat the problem, but often he or she will refer the patient to another health professional such as the ones described above, or to a surgeon.

SURGEONS

Surgeons are M.D.s, D.O.s, or D.P.M.s, and their patients are usually referred by another professional.

When a professional is needed, finding the one that best matches your particular need is very important.

BIBLIOGRAPHY

Adirim TA, Cheng TL (2003). Overview of injuries in the young athlete. Sports Med; 33(1): 75-81.

Baker MD, Bell RE (1991). The role of footwear in childhood injuries. Pediatr Emerg Care; 7(6): 353-355.

Barrett J, Bilisko T (1995). The role of shoes in the prevention of ankle sprains. Sports Med. 20(4): 277-280.

Basmajian JV, Bentzon JW (1954). An electromyographic study of certain muscles of the leg and foot in the standing position. Surg. Gynecol. Obstet. 98: 662-666. Abstr.

Brizuela G, Llana S, Ferrandis R, Garcia-Belenguer AC (1997). The influence of basketball shoes with increased ankle support on shock attenuation and performance in running and jumping. J. Sports Sci. 15(5): 505-515.

Bush RA, Brodine SK, Shaffer RA (2000). The association of blisters with musculoskeletal injuries in male marine recruits. J Am Podiatr Med Assoc; 90(4): 194-198.

Clanton TO, Butler JE, Eggert A (1986). Injuries to the metatarsophalangeal joints in athletes. Foot Ankle 7(3): 162-176.

DiGiovanni CW, Kuo R, Tejwani N et al. (2002). Isolated gastrocnemius tightness. J Bone Joint Surg Am; 84-A(6): 962-970.

Driano AN, Staheli L, Staheli LT (1998). Psychosocial development and corrective shoewear use in childhood. J Pediatr Orthop; 18(3): 346-349.

Gardner LI Jr, Dziados JE, Jones BH et al. (1988). Prevention of lower extremity stress fractures: a controlled trial of a shock absorbent insole. Am. J. Public Health 78(12): 1563-1567.

Grace TG, Skipper BJ, Newberry JC et al. (1988). Prophylactic knee braces and injury to the lower extremity. J. Bone Joint Surg. 70(3): 422-427.

Halperin JL (2002). Evaluation of patients with peripheral vascular disease. Thromb Res; 106(6): V303-311.

Hesse S, Luecke D, Jahnke MT, Mauritz KH (1996). Gait function in spastic hemiparetic patients walking barefoot, with firm shoes, and with ankle-foot orthosis. Int. J. Rehabil. Res; 19(2): 133-141.

Hogan MT, Staheli LT (2002). Arch height and lower limb pain: an adult civilian study. Foot Ankle Int; 23(1): 43-47.

Hopkins JT, Stencil R (2002). Ankle cryotherapy facilitates soleus function. J Orthop Sports Phys Ther; 32(12): 622-627.

Jorgensen U (1990). Body load in heel-strike running: the effect of a firm heel counter. Am. J. Sports Med. 18(2): 177-181.

Kanda F, Yagi E, Fukuda M et al. (1990). Elucidation of chemical compounds responsible for foot malodour. Br J Dermatol; 122(6): 771-776.

Kauranen K, Siira P, Vanharanta H (1997). The effect of strapping on the motor performance of the ankle and wrist joints. Scand J Med Sci Sports; 7(4): 238-243.

Knapik JJ, Reynolds KL, Duplantis KL, Jones BH (1995). Friction blisters. Pathophysiology, prevention and treatment. Sports Med; 20(3): 136-147.

Kogler GF, Veer FB, Verhulst SJ, et al. (2001). The effect of heel elevation on strain within the plantar aponeurosis: in vitro study. Foot Ankle Int; 22(5): 433-439.

Krivickas LS (1997). Anatomical factors associated with overuse sports injuries. Sports Med. 24(2): 132-146.

Leanderson J, Nemeth G, Eriksson E (1993). Ankle injuries in basketball players. Knee Surg. Sports Traumatol. Arthrosc; 1(3-4): 200-202.

Lin CC, Chang CT, Li TC, Kao CH (2002). Prediction of asymptomatically poor muscle perfusion of lower extremities in patients with type II diabetes mellitus using an objective radionuclide method. Endocr Res; 28(3): 265-270.

Matsusaka N, Yokoyama S, Tsurusaki T et al. (2001). Effect of ankle disk training combined with tactile stimulation to the leg and foot on functional instability of the ankle. Am J Sports Med; 29(1): 25-30

Menz HB, Lord SR (2001). The contribution of foot problems to mobility impairment and falls in community-dwelling older people. J Am Geriatr Soc; 49(12): 1651-1656.

Nurse MA, Nigg BM (2001). The effect of changes in foot sensation on plantar pressure and muscle activity. Clin Biomech (Bristol, Avon); 16(9): 719-727.

Perlman M, Leveille D, DeLeonibus J (1987). Inversion lateral ankle trauma: differential diagnosis, review of literature, and prospective studies. J. Foot. Surg; 26: 95-135.

Pinzur MS, Shields NN, Goelitz B, et al (1999). American Orthopaedic Foot and Ankle Society shoe survey of diabetic patients. Foot Ankle Int; 20(11): 703-707.

Ramsewak RS, Nair MG, Stommel M, Selanders L (2002). In vitro antagonistic activity of monoterpenes and their mixtures against 'toe nail fungus' pathogens. Phytother Res; 17(4): 376-379.

Rao UB, Joseph B (1992). The influence of footwear on the prevalence of flat foot. A survey of 2300 children. J Bone Joint Surg Br; 74(4): 525-527.

Robbins S, Gouw GJ, McClaran J, Waked E (1993). Protective sensation of the plantar aspect of the foot. Foot Ankle; 14(6): 347-52.

Robbins S, Hanna AM (1987). Running-related injury prevention through barefoot adaptations. Med. Sci. Sports Exerc; 19(2): 148-156.

Robbins S, Waked E (1997). Balance and vertical impact in sports: role of shoe sole materials. Arch. Phys. Med. Rehabil; 78(5): 463-467.

Robbins S, Waked E (1997). Hazard of deceptive advertising of athletic footwear. Br. J. Sports Med; 31(4): 299-303.

Robbins S, Waked E (1998). Factors associated with ankle injuries. Sports Med; 25(1): 63-72.

Robbins S, Waked E, Gouw GJ, McClaran J (1994). Athletic footwear affects balance in men. Br. J. Sports Med; 28(2): 117-122.

Robbins S, Waked E, McClaran J (1995). Proprioception and stability: foot position awareness as a function of age and footwear. Age Ageing; 24(1): 67-72.

Robbins S, Waked E, Rappel R (1995). Ankle taping improves proprioception before and after exercise in young men. Br. J. Sports Med; 29(4): 242-247.

Rovere GD, Clarke TJ, Yates CS, Burley K (1988). Retrospective comparison of taping and ankle stabilizers in preventing ankle injuries. Am. J. Sports Med; 16(3): 228-233.

Rovere GD, Haupt HA, Yates CS (1987). Prophylactic knee bracing in college football. Am. J. Sports Med; 15(2): 111-116.

Sachithanandam V, Joseph B (1995). The influence of footwear on the prevalence of flat foot. A survey of 1846 skeletally mature persons. J Bone Joint Surg Br; 77(2): 254-257.

Schuit D, Adrian M, Pidcoe P (1989). Effect of heel lifts on ground reaction force patterns in subjects with structural leg-length discrepancies. Phys Ther; 69(8): 663-670.

Springett K (2002). Introduction to some common cutaneous foot conditions and their management. J Tissue Viability; 12(3): 100-1, 104-107.

Staheli LT (1991). Shoes for children: a review. Pediatrics; 88(2): 371-375.

Staheli LT (1999). Planovalgus foot deformity. Current status. J Am Podiatr Med Assoc; 89(2): 94-99.

Swift CG (2001). Falls in late life and their consequences—implementing effective services. BMJ; 322: 855-857.

Teitz CC, Hermanson BK, Kronmal RA, Diehr PH (1987). Evaluation of the use of braces to prevent injury to the knee in collegiate football players. J. Bone Joint Surg; 69(1): 2-9.

Thonnard JL, Bragard D, Willems PA (1996). Stability of the braced ankle: a biomechanical investigation. Am. J. Sports Med; 24: 356-361.

Tomaro J, Burdett RG (1993). The effects of foot orthotics on the EMG activity of selected leg muscles during gait. J. Orthop. Sports Phys. Ther; 18(4): 532-536.

ENDNOTE

While writing about important topics such as fixing your feet, which can become a bit technical at times, it's also enjoyable to write in different prose. Below is a song I wrote following completion of my first proposal for this book. The words ring true despite not being able to include the music.

BAREFOOT IN AMERICA

Philip Maffetone

I walk out my door on a hot summer day.
And wanna test my freedom so I stay out to play.

I go anywhere I want with nothing on my feet.
To church, school, and restaurants, with everyone I meet.

> I go barefoot in America.
> Freedom everyday.
> Barefoot in America.
> Barefoot all the way.

They tell me not to enter here, they say I can't come in.
I ask them for a beer, when they say "no" I ask for gin.

I drive my car without my shoes, no law can stop me now.
I get those looks and I just muse, when some applaud I bow.

> Barefoot in America.
> Freedom everyday.
> Barefoot in America.
> Barefoot all the way.

I stop to see my lady friend in her shiny badge and blues.
I offer to bend down and take off her shoes.

I go anywhere I please with nothing on my feet.
I'm free here in America with everyone I meet.

> Barefoot in America
> Freedom everyday
> Barefoot in America
> Barefoot all the way.

© 2002 Philip Maffetone Volume I. Used with permission.

INDEX

Page numbers in boldface refer to illustrations.

DATE DUE

JAN 0 3 2005		
FEB 1 1 2005		
MAR 2 4 2005		
MAY 1 7 2005		
JUL 0 5 2005		
AUG 1 9 2005		
GAYLORD		PRINTED IN U.S.A.